Follicular Lymphoma

Editor

JONATHAN W. FRIEDBERG

HEMATOLOGY/ONCOLOGY CLINICS OF NORTH AMERICA

www.hemonc.theclinics.com

Consulting Editors
GEORGE P. CANELLOS
EDWARD J. BENZ Jr

August 2020 • Volume 34 • Number 4

ELSEVIER

1600 John F. Kennedy Boulevard • Suite 1800 • Philadelphia, Pennsylvania, 19103-2899

http://www.theclinics.com

HEMATOLOGY/ONCOLOGY CLINICS OF NORTH AMERICA Volume 34, Number 4
August 2020 ISSN 0889-8588, ISBN 13: 978-0-323-75438-5

Editor: Stacy Eastman
Developmental Editor: Julia McKenzie

Hematology/Oncology Clinics (ISSN 0889-8588) is published bimonthly by Elsevier Inc., 360 Park Avenue South, New York, NY 10010-1710. Months of issue are February, April, June, August, October, and December. Business and Editorial Offices: 1600 John F. Kennedy Blvd., Ste. 1800, Philadelphia, PA 19103–2899. Customer Service Office: 3251 Riverport Lane, Maryland Heights, MO 63043. Periodicals postage paid at New York, NY and at additional mailing offices. Subscription prices are $443.00 per year (domestic individuals), $876.00 per year (domestic institutions), $100.00 per year (domestic students/residents), $480.00 per year (Canadian individuals), $100.00 per year (Canadian students/residents), $1085.00 per year (Canadian institutions) $547.00 per year (international individuals), $1085.00 per year (international institutions), and $255.00 per year (international students/residents). International air speed delivery is included in all *Clinics* subscription prices. All prices are subject to change without notice. **POSTMASTER:** Send address changes to *Hematology/Oncology Clinics of North America*, Elsevier Health Sciences Division, Subscription Customer Service, 3251 Riverport Lane, Maryland Heights, MO 63043. Customer Service (orders, claims, online, change of address): Elsevier Health Sciences Division, Subscription **Customer Service, 3251 Riverport Lane, Maryland Heights, MO 63043. Tel: 1-800-654-2452 (U.S. and Canada); 314-447-8871 (outside U.S. and Canada). Fax: 314-447-8029. E-mail: journalscustomerservice-usa@elsevier.com (for print support); journalsonlinesupport-usa@elsevier.com (for online support)**.

Reprints. For copies of 100 or more, of articles in this publication, please contact the Commercial Reprints Department, Elsevier Inc., 360 Park Avenue South, New York, New York 10010-1710; Tel.: 212-633-3874, Fax: 212-633-3820, E-mail: reprints@elsevier.com.

Hematology/Oncology Clinics of North America is covered in *MEDLINE/PubMed (Index Medicus), EMBASE/ Excerpta Medica, and BIOSIS.*

Contributors

CONSULTING EDITORS

GEORGE P. CANELLOS, MD
William Rosenberg Professor of Medicine, Department of Medical Oncology, Dana-Farber Cancer Institute, Boston, Massachusetts, USA

EDWARD J. BENZ Jr, MD
Professor, Pediatrics, Richard and Susan Smith Professor, Medicine, Professor, Genetics, Harvard Medical School, President and CEO Emeritus, Office of the President, Dana-Farber Cancer Institute, Boston, Massachusetts, USA

EDITOR

JONATHAN W. FRIEDBERG, MD, MMSc
Samuel Durand Professor of Medicine and Oncology, Director, Wilmot Cancer Institute, University of Rochester School of Medicine, Rochester, New York, USA

AUTHORS

PAUL M. BARR, MD
James P. Wilmot Cancer Institute, University of Rochester Medical Center, Rochester, New York, USA

CARLA CASULO, MD
Associate Professor, Medicine and Oncology, Wilmot Cancer Institute, Rochester, New York, USA

JAMES R. CERHAN, MD, PhD
Professor and Chair, Department of Health Sciences Research, Mayo Clinic, Rochester, Minnesota, USA

COLLIN K. CHIN, MBBS
Fellow, Department of Lymphoma/Myeloma, The University of Texas MD Anderson Cancer Center, Houston, Texas, USA

JONATHON B. COHEN, MD, MS
Associate Professor, Department of Hematology and Medical Oncology, Winship Cancer Institute of Emory University, Atlanta, Georgia, USA

JUDE FITZGIBBON, BA, PhD
Centre for Cancer Genomics and Computational Biology, Barts Cancer Institute, Queen Mary University of London, London, United Kingdom

CIARA L. FREEMAN, MB BCh, MSc, FRCPathUK, FRCPC
Assistant Professor, BC Cancer Centre for Lymphoid Cancer, The University of British Columbia, Vancouver, British Columbia, Canada

CAMILLE GOLFIER, MD
Assistant Professor, Department of Hematology, Hospices Civils de Lyon, Hôpital Lyon-Sud, Pierre-Bénite France and Université de Lyon, Université Claude Bernard, Faculté de Médecine Lyon-Sud, Oullins, France

AJAY K. GOPAL, MD
Division of Medical Oncology, Department of Medicine, University of Washington, Clinical Research Division, Fred Hutchinson Cancer Research Center, Seattle, Washington, USA

BRAD S. KAHL, MD
Professor, Department of Medicine, Washington University School of Medicine, St Louis, Missouri, USA

EMIL A. KUMAR, BA, BM, BCh
Centre for Cancer Genomics and Computational Biology, Barts Cancer Institute, Queen Mary University of London, London, United Kingdom

JODI J. LIPOF, MD
James P. Wilmot Cancer Institute, University of Rochester Medical Center, Rochester, New York, USA

RYAN C. LYNCH, MD
Assistant Professor, Division of Medical Oncology, Department of Medicine, University of Washington, Assistant Member, Clinical Research Division, Fred Hutchinson Cancer Research Center, Seattle, Washington, USA

SILVIA MONTOTO, MD
Consultant Haemato-Oncologist, Department of Haemato-Oncology, St Bartholomew's Hospital, London, United Kingdom

FRANCK MORSCHHAUSER, MD, PhD
Univ. Lille, CHU Lille, ULR 7365 - GRITA - Groupe de Recherche Sur les Formes Injectables et les Technologies Associees, Lille, France

LORETTA J. NASTOUPIL, MD
Associate Professor, Department of Lymphoma/Myeloma, The University of Texas MD Anderson Cancer Center, Houston, Texas, USA

JESSICA OKOSUN, MB, BChir, PhD
Clinical Senior Lecturer, Centre for Haemato-Oncology, Barts Cancer Institute, Queen Mary University of London, John Vane Science Centre, London, United Kingdom

ANAND A. PATEL, MD
Department of Medicine, Section of Hematology-Oncology, The University of Chicago, Chicago, Illinois, USA

GILLES SALLES, MD, PhD
Department Head and Professor of Medicine, Department of Hematology, Hospices Civils de Lyon, Lyon-Sud, Pierre-Bénite France and Université de Lyon, Université Claude Bernard, Faculté de Médecine Lyon-Sud, Oullins, France

LAURIE H. SEHN, MD, MPH
Clinical Professor, BC Cancer Centre for Lymphoid Cancer, The University of British Columbia, Vancouver, British Columbia, Canada

SONALI M. SMITH, MD, FASCO
Elwood V. Jensen Professor of Medicine, Interim Chief, Section of Hematology/Oncology, Director, Lymphoma Program, Department of Medicine, The University of Chicago, Chicago, Illinois, USA

LOIC YSEBAERT, MD, PhD
Service d'Hematologie, Institut Universitaire du Cancer de Toulouse-Oncopole, Center for Cancer Research of Toulouse (CRCT), Inserm UMR1037, IUC-Toulouse-Oncopole, Toulouse, France

Contents

Follicular lymphoma (FL) is a common indolent lymphoma subtype in Western countries. FL incidence increases with age, and shows considerable variation by race/ethnicity and geography. In the United States and France, FL incidence has been stable since 2000, whereas in other Western and Asian countries it has been increasing. Five-year relative survival rates have been increasing in Western and Asian countries. Progress on identifying FL-specific risk factors has accelerated with the implementation of the InterLymph nested classification and the availability of larger epidemiologic studies and pooled analyses. Identification of risk factors for FL requires further research.

Follicular lymphoma comprises approximately 20-30% of all cases of B-cell lymphomas. Median survival has improved significantly in the modern era. Prognostic factors include histologic grade, cytogenetics, molecular mutations, the tumor microenvironment, and tumor burden. Clinical prognostic indices are available and increasingly incorporate genetic information. Prognostic factors also arise during the course of treatment. Early progression within 24 months of initial chemoimmunotherapy is an adverse prognostic marker of inferior survival. Other high-risk populations include those with double refractory disease or those with high risk of transformation to diffuse large B-cell lymphoma.

Patients with early stage follicular lymphoma frequently have prolonged overall survival and 40% may remain progression-free 20 years after receiving radiation therapy alone. Thus, such an approach is often considered in this population. Patients with advanced-stage disease but low tumor burden do not achieve a survival benefit by initiation treatment but early therapy with rituximab can improve quality of life and prolong time until need for further treatment and/or chemotherapy. Patients with advanced-stage follicular lymphoma who have low tumor burden should be managed in a personalized fashion taking into account individual feeling regarding treatment, toxicity, and long-term goals.

requiring therapy, and is approved in relapsed/refractory FL. We review the biology supporting the rationale for adequate inhibitory receptor/ligand pathways targeting the tissue immune microenvironment of FL cells, and potential immunomodulating combinations to replace CIT in the near future.

Chemoimmunotherapy is the standard frontline treatment for symptomatic or high tumor burden follicular lymphoma. Better understanding of the molecular mechanisms of lymphomagenesis has led to the development of drugs targeting these pathways. The phosphatidylinositol-3-kinase pathway is an important signaling pathway in B-cell lymphomas. Three drugs in this class have received FDA approval. We describe the efficacy and toxicities of phosphatidylinositol-3-kinase inhibitors. Response rates in highly refractory disease are high, demonstrate few long-term remissions, and have high long-term toxicity. Early data on dosing and combination strategies are promising and may change how we use these agents in the coming years.

Follicular lymphoma is the most common indolent non-Hodgkin lymphoma. Although median overall survival rates exceed 12 years with rituximab, follicular lymphoma remains largely incurable. The growing understanding of the molecular drivers of lymphomagenesis and the tumor microenvironment have led to novel therapies. Prognostic markers have identified a subset of patients with chemoresistant and/or refractory disease-associated poor outcomes. We identify the patients with follicular lymphoma in need of novel therapies, describe the drivers of lymphomagenesis and importance of the tumor microenvironment, and summarize the novel agents under investigation in relapsed/refractory and upfront follicular lymphoma.

Follicular lymphoma is the most common subtype of indolent non-Hodgkin lymphoma. Although a majority of patients have a favorable prognosis, a subset of patients experiences early treatment failure. Progression of disease within 24 months of initial chemoimmunotherapy is associated with inferior survival. The biology of early progression is the subject of ongoing study and depends on the unique genetic composition of neoplastic cells and their interaction with a complex tumor microenvironment. Clinicogenetic prognostic indices have been developed to identify high-risk patients. Several have been validated but are limited in identifying those at risk for early treatment failure.

Histologic transformation of follicular lymphoma remains the leading cause of follicular lymphoma-related mortality in the rituximab era. Both the diverse timing of transformation and heterogeneity in associated genomic events suggest that histologic transformation may itself comprise distinct disease entities. Successive indolent and transformation episodes occur by divergent clonal evolution from an inferred common progenitor cell, representing a potential therapeutic target. Existing biological knowledge largely pre-dates anti-CD20 therapy, and further prospective validation is essential. Inclusion of transformation cases in clinical trials incorporating biomarker discovery, and an integrated understanding of the genetic and microenvironmental factors underpinning transformation, may unearth renewed clinical opportunities.

Histologic transformation from follicular lymphoma to aggressive lymphoma historically had a poor prognosis. Routine use of anti-CD20 antibody rituximab has changed the landscape of follicular lymphoma (FL) such that outcomes are improved in select patients, similar to de-novo diffuse large B-cell lymphoma. Several biological and clinical biomarkers can predict risk of transformation, and ongoing research is improving understanding of the biology surrounding the transformation process. This review provides an overview of risk factors, prognosis, and treatment of histologic transformation of FL.

HEMATOLOGY/ONCOLOGY CLINICS OF NORTH AMERICA

SERIES OF RELATED INTEREST

Surgical Oncology Clinics of North America
https://www.surgonc.theclinics.com/

THE CLINICS ARE AVAILABLE ONLINE!
Access your subscription at:
www.theclinics.com

Preface

Toward a Cure for Follicular Lymphoma

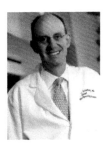

Jonathan W. Friedberg, MD, MMSc
Editor

In 1984, Horning and Rosenberg published a seminal paper describing the natural history of follicular lymphoma (then also referred to as nodular poorly differentiated lymphocytic lymphoma) emphasizing the incidence of spontaneous regressions and histological transformation over time, the lack of benefit of early therapeutic intervention, and the incurable nature of the disease with a median overall survival of 11 years. They concluded that "an increased understanding of the cause and regulation of these low-grade B-cell neoplasms and their potential manipulation by new therapeutic approaches offers exciting avenues for research and should be pursued."[1]

As evidenced by this issue of *Hematology/Oncology Clinics of North America*, these remarks could not have been more prescient. Our therapeutic armamentarium is now dramatically expanded, beginning with the approval of rituximab in 1997, followed by other agents, including lenalidomide, PI-3 kinase inhibitors, novel antibody and immunotherapy constructs, and other signaling pathway inhibitors. Our understanding of the appropriate application of chemoimmunotherapy combinations and the ongoing controversies about role of maintenance therapies have dramatically improved response durations for most patients. The initial observation of spontaneous regressions led to enthusiasm for the application of cellular therapies in this disease, including allogeneic stem cell transplantation and, more recently, CAR-T cell therapy. Taken together, these insights have allowed the median overall survival to now greatly exceed 20 years for advanced stage presentations, meaning many or most patients diagnosed with follicular lymphoma will die with, rather than of, follicular lymphoma.

Yet, important questions about managing this disease remain. Histologic transformation to more aggressive histology remains an important cause of morbidity and mortality for patients with follicular lymphoma. We have greatly improved our understanding of the clonal dynamics that contribute to histological transformation, and indeed the truly complex biology—intrinsic to the malignant B cell as well as the

Hematol Oncol Clin N Am 34 (2020) xiii–xiv
https://doi.org/10.1016/j.hoc.2020.05.001
0889-8588/20/© 2020 Published by Elsevier Inc.

hemonc.theclinics.com

tumor microenvironment—at diagnosis and over the disease course. Harnessing this understanding to prevent transformation remains an elusive goal. The epidemiology of follicular lymphoma has revealed an increased incidence over the past 35 years without clear understanding why in most cases, although molecular insights should ultimately provide strategies for prevention. A relatively small subset of patients—difficult to identify at diagnosis—have a more aggressive disease course with substantially increased mortality; this is currently the top priority for clinical trials by US National Clinical Trials Network.[2]

I'll close with the biggest question: can we cure this disease? We already know that more than 40% of patients remain in remission 10 years after initial treatment with R-CHOP; it is likely a subset of these patients will not relapse in their lifetimes.[3] Given numerous classes of therapeutic agents, our understanding of the heterogeneous nature of this disease, and ongoing research incorporating both tumor and microenvironmental biology, I'm optimistic that a cure for most patients is on the horizon. The articles in this issue, following in the footsteps of Horning and Rosenberg, lay the groundwork for this imperative.

Jonathan W. Friedberg, MD, MMSc
Wilmot Cancer Institute
University of Rochester School of Medicine
601 Elmwood Avenue, Box 704
Rochester, NY 14610, USA

E-mail address:
Jonathan_Friedberg@urmc.rochester.edu

REFERENCES

1. Horning SJ, Rosenberg SA. The natural history of initially untreated low-grade non-Hodgkin's lymphomas. N Engl J Med 1984;311:1471–5.
2. Maddocks K, Barr PM, Cheson BD, et al. Recommendations for clinical trial development in follicular lymphoma. J Natl Cancer Inst 2017;109(3):djw255.
3. Friedberg JW. Progress in advanced-stage follicular lymphoma. J Clin Oncol 2018; 36:2363–5.

Epidemiology of Follicular Lymphoma

James R. Cerhan, MD, PhD

KEYWORDS

- Epidemiology • Follicular lymphoma • Risk • Genetics • Infection • Environmental
- Prevention

KEY POINTS

- An estimated 14,000 cases of follicular lymphoma (FL) were diagnosed in the United States in 2016; FL incidence is slightly higher in men, increases steeply with age, and is highest in non-Hispanic white people.
- FL incidence shows geographic variation, has been stable in the United States and France since 2000, but has been increasing in other Western and Asian countries.
- Five-year relative survival rates in the United States range from 80% to 90% across sex and major racial/ethnic groups; relative survival rates have been increasing since 2000 in the United States and other Western and Asian countries.
- Beyond family history of non-Hodgkin lymphoma, genetic loci, and Sjögren syndrome, there are no established risk factors for FL, although there are promising leads related to atopy, certain infections, anthropometrics, hair dye, recreational sun exposure, smoking, and alcohol use.

INTRODUCTION

Follicular lymphoma (FL) is one of the most common indolent non-Hodgkin lymphoma (NHL) subtype in Western countries. Although understanding of the epidemiology of NHL subtypes has been hampered by changes in classification over time, this situation has greatly improved since the implementation of the World Health Organization (WHO) classification for hematologic and lymphoma tissues in 2001[1] and the nested classification of lymphoid neoplasms for epidemiologic research from the International Lymphoma Epidemiology Consortium (InterLymph) in 2007.[2] The diagnosis of FL has high concordance between referral and expert review (85.5%),[3] and, unlike many NHL subtypes, FL has good agreement between the InterLymph classification and the historical Working formulation (88.9%),[2] allowing for a longer time range of epidemiologic studies that can address FL time trends and risk factors. Nevertheless, a historical focus on NHL overall and a lack of NHL subtype information in epidemiologic studies before the 1980s, along with limited sample sizes, has hampered progress. A

Department of Health Sciences Research, Mayo Clinic, 200 1st Street Southwest, Rochester, MN 55905, USA
E-mail address: cerhan.james@mayo.edu

Hematol Oncol Clin N Am 34 (2020) 631–646
https://doi.org/10.1016/j.hoc.2020.02.001
0889-8588/20/© 2020 Elsevier Inc. All rights reserved.

comprehensive review of the epidemiology of NHL was recently published,[4] and this review focuses on FL descriptive epidemiology as well as analytical epidemiology based on larger and more definitive studies, especially meta-analyses and pooled analyses.

DESCRIPTIVE EPIDEMIOLOGY
Incidence

In 2016, an estimated 13,960 cases were diagnosed in the United States, representing 12.4% of mature NHLs.[5] For the later part of the twentieth century, NHL rates were rapidly increasing in Western countries and then stabilized around 2000.[4] FL incidence in the United States increased from 1992 to 2001.[6] Using data from the US Surveillance, Epidemiology, and End Results (SEER) program,[7] the age-adjusted incidence rate (using the US year 2000 as the standard population) for FL from 2000 to 2016 was 3.5 per 100,000, and was 1.2 times higher in men (3.9) than in women (3.3). The incidence of FL increases sharply with age (**Fig. 1**). Rates were highest in non-Hispanic white people (4.1), followed by Hispanic people of all races (2.9), then non-Hispanic black people (2.4), American-Indian/Alaska Natives (1.7), and Asian or Pacific Islanders (1.7). As shown in **Fig. 2**, from 2000 to 2016 the incidence rates have been steady for all ethnicity/race and gender groups with the exception of statistically

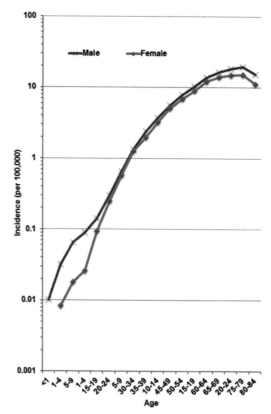

Fig. 1. Incidence rates by age group for FL. SEER program, 18 registries (SEER18), United States, 2000 to 2016.

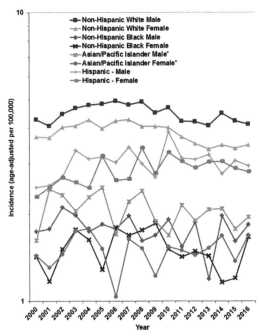

Fig. 2. Age-adjusted incidence rates for FL by gender and race/ethnicity. The asterisks indicate non-Hispanic. SEER18, United States, 2000 to 2016.

significant (P<.05) decreases for non-Hispanic white women (annual percentage change, −0.98%) and increases for Hispanic women (+1.01%).

There are fewer data to make international comparisons, but, in a large international pathology study of the relative frequencies of NHL subtypes from 24 countries, FL accounted for a higher percentage in developed countries (25.5%) compared with developing countries (15.3%).[8] Compared with age-standardized incidence rates in the United States for FL (3.5), rates were lower in Australia for 1997 to 2006 (3.1),[9] Europe for 2000 to 2002 (2.2),[10] the United Kingdom for 2004 to 2012 (2.8),[11] Singapore for 2008 to 2012 (1.0),[12] and Japan for 2008 (1.1),[13] acknowledging differences in cancer registration, time frames, and standard populations. Age-adjusted FL rates were also slightly higher for women than men in Europe and the United Kingdom, but not in the United States, Australia, Singapore, or Japan. Differences in age-standardized rates for FL by ethnicity were also observed in the United Kingdom for 2001 to 2007, with the highest rates in white people (1.6) then South Asians (1.2), black people (0.6), and Chinese (0.6).[14] FL incidence rates stabilized in France for 2000 to 2009,[15] whereas they were still increasing in Australia for 1997 to 2008,[9] Singapore for 1998 to 2012,[12] and Japan for 1993 to 2008.[13] The world age-standardized rates (per 100,000) of FL in Chinese migrants from Hong Kong to British Columbia (1.21) was closer to that of Hong Kong (1.66) than that of non-Chinese in British Columbia (2.97),[16] suggesting potential genetic differences in susceptibility not affected by migration to a new environment with higher FL rates.

Survival and Mortality

The 5-year relative survival rate for FL, which accounts for competing causes of mortality, is summarized in **Fig. 3** from the SEER program (18 registries) for cases

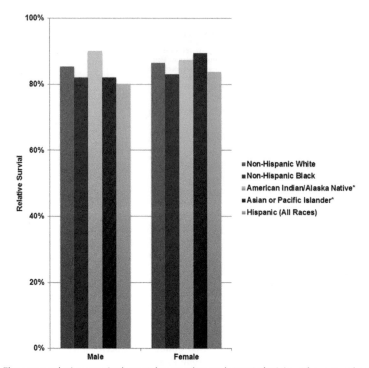

Fig. 3. Five-year relative survival rates by gender and race/ethnicity. The asterisks indicate non-Hispanic. SEER18, United States, 2000 to 2016.

diagnosed from 2000 to 2016 by race/ethnicity and gender.[7] Rates ranged from 80% to 90%, were similar by gender, and were highest for male American Indians/Alaska Natives (90.2%) and lowest for Hispanic men (80.2%). The 5-year relative survival rate for FL in the EUROCARE-5 (European Cancer Registry Based Study on Survival and Care of Cancer Patients-5) study[17] of 20 countries increased between 2000 to 2002 (64.1%) and 2003 to 2005 (69.0%) and then to 2006 to 2008 (74.3%), whereas in the United Kingdom[11] it was 86.5% for cases diagnosed 2004 to 2012. In Singapore,[12] 5-year age-standardized relative survival for FL increased between 1998 to 2002 (43.8%) and 2003 to 2007 (64.9%) and 2008 to 2012 (82.3%). In the SEER program, overall survival rates for FL improved in all age and sex groups for the period 2001 to 2009 compared with 1992 to 2000.[18] Similarly, overall and relative survival improved from 2000 to 2010 in Sweden in all age and sex groups, particularly elderly women, and correlated with the adoption of first-line rituximab use.[19]

Using a landmark analysis, patients with FL who had a progression, relapse, or retreatment within 12 months of diagnosis had poor subsequent overall survival compared with an age-matched and sex-matched background population (standardized mortality ratio = 3.72; 95% confidence interval [CI], 2.78 to 4.88), whereas patients who did not have any of these events in the 12 months after diagnosis had no added mortality beyond the background population; for immunochemotherapy-treated patients, this landmark occurred at 24 months after diagnosis.[20] These results emphasize the clinical importance of early failures, whereas patients achieving event-free status at 12 or 24 months can expect a normal life expectancy.

Although relative survival has been increasing since 2000, lymphoma remains the leading cause of death in the first decade after diagnosis in patients with FL treated in the rituximab era, with a cumulative risk of mortality of 10.3% at 10 years (and 13.3% when combined with treatment-related mortality).[21] In contrast, the cumulative risk of mortality as a result of non–lymphoma-related causes was 5.1% at 10 years. Notable, the 10-year cumulative risk of lymphoma or treatment-related mortality for patients with an event within 24 months of diagnosis was 36.1% (compared with 6.7% for patients achieving event-free survival at 24 months) and after transformation was 45.9% (compared with 8.1% for patients who did not transform), emphasizing the importance of these events in driving poor outcomes in FL.

Mortalities for FL are not available, because NHL subtype information is rarely recorded on death certificates. Using SEER and other population data, Howlander and colleagues[22] showed that overall NHL mortalities increased from 1975 to 1997, and then decreased from 1998 to 2011, and that incidence-based mortalities (an approach to link NHL subtype incidence data with mortality data) for FL began to decline 5.3% per year after 1997. In 2011, an estimated 11% of NHL deaths in the United States were caused by FL.[22]

PRECURSORS

The t(14;18) translocation, giving rise to a *BCL2-IGH* fusion, is a genetic hallmark of FL (>85% of patients with FL have the translocation). It can be been detected at low levels in 50% to 70% of presumably normal adults, and higher levels of circulating t(14;18) cells (>1 in 10,000 blood cells) is associated with a 23-fold higher risk of developing FL (95% CI, 9.98–67.3).[23] Even with this strong association, the high prevalence of the biomarker relative to the low incidence of FL suggests the t(14;18) event is necessary but not sufficient for follicular lymphomagenesis.

FAMILY HISTORY AND GENETIC SUSCEPTIBILITY

In the InterLymph Subtypes Project, a family history of NHL was associated with a 1.99-fold increased risk of FL (95% CI, 1.55–2.54) and this association was not attenuated by adjustment for potential confounding factors.[24] This risk estimate aligns with data from a pooled analysis of 5 Nordic registries from 1955 to 2010 (standardized incidence ratio [SIR] = 1.6; 95% CI, 1.4 to 2.0). Risk of FL was also increased in persons with a first-degree relative with FL (SIR = 2.1; 95% CI, 1.3–3.4), diffuse large B-cell lymphoma (DLBCL) (SIR = 2.6; 95% CI, 1.7–3.6), small lymphocytic lymphoma (SLL) (SIR = 3.6; 95% CI, 1.0–9.1), mantle cell lymphoma (MCL) (SIR = 2.6; 95% CI, 0.9–6.1),[25] HL (odds ratio [OR] = 1.47; 95% CI, 0.90–2.40),[24] multiple myeloma (OR = 1.93; 95% CI, 1.06–3.51),[24] and chronic lymphocytic leukemia (CLL) (OR = 1.6; 95% CI, 0.87–2.8).[26] Although familial aggregation represents both shared genetic and environmental factors, the findings to date suggest that the associations with family history are not strongly confounded by nongenetic risk factors.[27] Furthermore, there seems to be shared cause across multiple subtypes, with many subtypes showing a stronger association with a family history for that specific subtype, suggesting a role for subtype-specific genetic factors.[27]

Genetic epidemiology studies are used to identify genetic loci. Linkage studies in families are most commonly used to identify genes with major susceptibility effects (eg, mendelian), but there are no linkage studies of FL or most major NHL subtypes.[27] The lack of major genes in FL and other common NHL subtypes may be caused by underpowered studies and the complexity of accurate phenotyping of NHL subtypes over time, but alternatively raises the hypothesis that multiple, low-risk to moderate-risk variants that are common in the population (ie, >5% minor allele frequency) may be more relevant in lymphoma causes than single, highly penetrant variants that are very rare.[28] To identify common genetic variants, the case-control study design is most commonly used, and either evaluates candidate genes (hypothesis driven) or the entire genome simultaneously via an agnostic (hypothesis-free) genome-wide association study (GWAS) approach.[27] Before GWAS, there were a large number of studies evaluating candidate genes with risk of FL, but most of the studies failed to replicate for a variety of reasons.[29] In the largest GWAS, of more than 2100 FL cases, the human leukocyte antigen (HLA) region showed a striking association with FL, with the top single nucleotide polymorphism (SNP) at 6p21.32 (rs12195582) reaching $P = 5.36 \times 10^{-100}$, which is far exceeds the GWAS significance level of 5×10^{-8}.[30] After imputing HLA alleles and amino acids (AAs), the strongest signal mapped to 4 linked DRβ1 multiallelic AAs at positions 11, 13, 28, and 30, which reside in the peptide binding cleft and affect several binding pockets in DRβ1. Because these are key positions that affect allelic binding, these results suggest an important role for DRβ1 peptide presentation in the cause of FL. After accounting for this locus, 2 additional independent, genome-wide signals were identified in HLA class II (rs17203612) and class I (rs3130437, near *HLA-C*). Outside of the HLA region, loci were identified at 11q23.3 (near *CRCX5*), 11q24.3 (near *ETS1*), 3q28 (in *LPP*), 18q21.33 (near *BCL2*), and 8q24.21 (near *PVT1*). These genes all link B-cell biology to follicular lymphomagenesis. In the context of GWAS of other lymphoma subtypes, FL shares loci (although specific SNP results vary) at 6q21.32-33 with DLBCL, CLL, Hodgkin lymphoma (HL), marginal zone lymphoma (MZL), and NKTCL; 8q24 with DLBCL, CLL, and HL; 3q28 with CLL; and 18q21.33 with CLL.[28] These results parallel the family study data, supporting a genetic architecture of risk across subtypes as well as for specific subtypes.

MEDICAL HISTORY RISK FACTORS
Infections

The International Agency for Research on Cancer (IARC) has classified Epstein-Barr virus, hepatitis C virus (HCV), human immunodeficiency virus (HIV) type 1, Kaposi sarcoma herpes virus, human T-cell lymphotropic virus type 1, and *Helicobacter pylori* as carcinogenic to humans (group 1) with sufficient evidence that they cause certain types of lymphoma in humans, but only HCV has shown an association with FL.[31] HCV infection was associated with FL (OR = 2.73; 95% CI, 2.20–3.38) in a meta-analysis of 542 FL cases and 4041 controls,[32] and this association was also observed in a large SEER-Medicare case-control study (OR = 1.88; 95% CI, 1.17–3.02).[33] However, in an InterLymph pooled analysis of 1181 FL cases and 6269 controls, HCV seropositivity was not associated with FL (OR = 1.02; 95% CI, 0.65–1.60).[34] Treatment of HCV can induce remission of FL.[35]

In a 2009 evaluation, IARC judged that there was only limited evidence of a causal link of hepatitis B virus (HBV) with NHL,[36] although, in a more recent meta-analysis of 17 case-control and 5 cohort studies (>40,000 NHL cases), HBV infection was associated with an increased risk of NHL overall (OR = 2.24; 95% CI, 1.80–2.78), but, for FL, risk was only increased in studies from countries with high HBV prevalence (OR = 1.66; 95% CI, 1.02–2.70).[37]

Transplant

Solid organ transplant includes an early, intense induction phase of immunosuppression followed by a later maintenance phase and long-term chronic immune dysfunction. In a large cohort, solid organ transplant recipients had a 6-fold overall excess risk of NHL compared with the general population (SIR = 6.2; 95% CI, 5.9–6.5).[38] The excess risk was associated with a distinct spectrum of NHL subtypes (eg, DLBCL, Burkitt, and several T-cell lymphomas) that did not include indolent subtypes, including FL (SIR = 0.9; 95% CI, 0.7–1.3).

Autoimmunity and Atopy

In an InterLymph pooling project,[39] risk of FL was associated with Sjögren syndrome (OR = 3.91, 95% CI, 1.39–11.0), particularly secondary Sjögren syndrome (OR = 7.55; 95% CI, 1.75–32.7), but not other autoimmune disorders, including ulcerative colitis, type 1 diabetes, celiac disease, and systemic lupus erythematosus. Sjögren syndrome was also strongly associated with MZL (OR = 30.6) and DLBCL (OR = 8.92), suggesting potential shared pathogenesis. In the SEER-Medicare NHL case-control study, FL was associated with rheumatoid arthritis (OR = 1.3; 95% CI, 1.1–1.5), autoimmune hemolytic anemia (OR = 3.4; 95% CI, 1.4–8.2), and aplastic anemia (OR = 2.4; 95% CI, 1.1–5.2); was only weakly associated with Sjögren syndrome (OR = 1.3; 95% CI, 0.7–2.2); and was not associated with 22 other autoimmune conditions.[40]

A history of atopic disorders was inversely associated with FL (OR = 0.87; 95% 0.80–0.94), which was not confounded by other FL risk factors.[24] Inverse associations were observed for allergy (excluding drug allergy), food allergy, asthma, and hay fever (ORs, 0.79–0.88), but not eczema. However, the association of allergies and FL was null in the multiethnic cohort study (hazard ratio = 0.97; 95% CI, 0.64–1.47), raising some concern echoed more broadly in the NHL literature of reverse causality underlying this putative association.[41]

Immune Markers

Biomarkers of immune function, particularly circulating cytokine and chemokines, provide insight into lymphomagenesis. Although most studies have not reported subtype-specific NHL results, a meta-analysis of 4 general-population, HIV-negative cohort studies found positive associations of soluble CD30 (OR = 3.78 for greater than reference level; 95% CI, 2.50–5.72) and soluble CD27 (OR = 1.77; 95% CI, 1.04–2.09) with FL risk.[42] These soluble forms of tumor necrosis factor receptors are markers of B-cell activation, supporting a mechanistic role for chronic B-cell activation even at the subclinical level.

Hormonal and Reproductive

Unlike most NHL subtypes with a higher male sex ratio, in FL this is much smaller or even reversed, raising causal hypotheses related to hormonal and reproductive factors. In an InterLymph pooled analysis, FL risk was inversely associated with number of pregnancies (trend OR = 0.88; 95% CI, 0.81–0.96) and was positively associated with hormonal contraception use (OR = 1.30; 95% CI, 1.04–1.63), with higher risks for the latter when use started after age 21 years, use was less than 5 years, or use stopped more than 20 years before diagnosis.[43] There were no associations with menstrual history or other details of reproductive history. Postmenopausal hormone therapy (HT) was inversely associated with FL risk (OR = 0.82; 95% CI, 0.66–1.01) in an InterLymph pooled analysis, particularly for current use or later age at initiation.[44] Type of HT was not available, although, when stratified by history of hysterectomy, the inverse association for FL was only observed in women with an intact uterus. In contrast with case-control studies, cohort studies have generally found no or increased FL risk with HT, and, in the 13-year follow-up of the randomized portion of the Women's Health Initiative, unopposed estrogen or estrogen plus progestin was not associated with FL risk.[45]

Other Medical Exposures

Type 2 diabetes mellitus was not associated with FL in a meta-analysis of 4 studies.[46] Although risk of B-cell NHL increases after use of chemotherapy or radiotherapy for cancer treatment, most cases are aggressive subtypes and there are no risk estimates for FL.[47] Radiation after solid organ cancer was not associated with risk of FL, with the possible exception of radiotherapy for thyroid cancer (Relative Risk [RR] = 4.38; 95% CI, 1.40–13.7).[48] History of blood transfusion was not associated with FL risk in a meta-analysis of case-control and cohort studies.[49] In an InterLymph pooled analysis of 13 case-control studies, blood transfusion was inversely associated with FL in both men (OR = 0.70; 95% CI, 0.56–0.87) and women (OR = 0.77; 95% CI, 0.64–0.92)[50] and was not confounded by FL-specific risk factors.[24] The unexpected inverse association lacks a compelling causal explanation.[50]

OCCUPATIONAL AND ENVIRONMENTAL RISK FACTORS

In an InterLymph pooled analysis of 10 case-control studies (including 2140 FL cases), none of the 25 a priori defined occupational groups was associated with FL risk, although there were increased risks associated with specific occupations, including spray-painter (except construction) (OR = 2.67; 95% CI, 1.36–5.25) and greater than 10 years of employment as a medical doctor (OR = 2.23; 95% CI, 1.17–4.26), and decreased risks associated with employment as bakers/millers (OR = 0.54; 95% CI, 0.30–0.99) and university and higher education teachers (OR = 0.62; 95% CI, 0.44–0.89).[51] The few studies of pesticide exposure have either not reported FL-specific results or have had very small numbers. In a pooled analysis of 4 case-control studies on lymphoma risk and organophosphate and carbamate insecticide use, only malathion use was associated with FL (OR = 1.58; 95% CI, 1.11–2.27),[52] but this was not seen in a large meta-analysis[53] or pooled analysis of cohort studies.[54] In a systematic review and meta-analysis, only a DDT (dichlorodiphenyltrichloroethane) and FL association was identified (OR = 1.5; 95% CI, 1.0–2.4),[53] whereas in a pooled analysis of cohort studies of more than 300,000 agricultural workers (and 214 incident FL cases), none of the 14 pesticide chemical groups or 33 individual active ingredients were associated with FL.[54]

In an InterLymph pooling project, any use of hair dye was associated with increased risk of FL among women (OR = 1.3; 95% CI, 1.0–1.6), particularly for women who began using hair dye before 1980 (OR = 1.4; 95% CI, 1.1–1.9), where there were associations with duration of use for permanent, dark, and light color dyes as well as with cumulative use.[55] For women who started using hair dyes in 1980 or later, duration of use was only associated with use of permanent and dark-colored dyes. It is not clear whether these patterns reflect long-term usage or a change in dye formulations in the early 1980s.[4] Work as a hairdresser has not been associated with FL risk.[51]

FL risk was inversely associated with recreational sun exposure (OR = 0.73 for highest vs lowest quartile; 95% CI, 0.62–0.86) in an InterLymph pooled analysis,[56] and this association was not confounded by other FL risk factors.[24] A meta-analysis that also included cohort studies reported a slightly weaker association (RR = 0.78; 95% CI, 0.70–0.88) but no association with dietary vitamin D intake or serum/plasma 25-hydroxyvitamin D,[57] leaving immunomodulation by sun exposure as a more promising mechanism.[4]

LIFESTYLE AND BEHAVIORAL RISK FACTORS
Smoking

Cigarette smoking was not associated with FL overall in 2 large meta-analyses,[58,59] although in 1 meta-analysis[58] increased risk of FL in former female smokers was observed but only in case-control studies (OR = 1.33; 95% CI, 1.07–1.66). In an Inter-Lymph pooled analysis, cigarette smoking was associated with FL risk in women (OR = 1.22; 95% CI, 1.09–1.37) but not men (OR = 0.98; 95% CI, 0.87–1.10; P hetero-geneity = 0.004), and this was limited to current smokers and was more strongly related to duration than frequency of cigarettes smoked.[24] A large cohort study not in the meta-analyses also found that female current smokers had an increased risk of FL (RR = 2.13; 95% CI, 1.20–3.77) that was not apparent among former female smokers or men.[60]

Alcohol

Alcohol drinkers had a lower risk of FL (OR = 0.80; 95% CI, 0.69–0.92) in a meta-analysis of 21 case-control and 8 cohort studies, which was observed for NHL overall (OR = 0.85; 95% CI, 0.79–0.91) and for most major subtypes except CLL/SLL.[61] An updated meta-analysis of only cohort studies also found an inverse association of alcohol use with FL (OR = 0.85; 95% CI, 0.78–0.93) and no strong association with type of alcohol.[62] In the InterLymph Subtypes Project, history of alcohol use was inversely associated with FL among women (OR = 0.79; 95% CI, 0.68–0.91) but not men (OR = 0.95; 95% CI, 0.80–1.12), and there was no clear pattern with type of alcohol, duration, number of drinks, or cumulative alcohol consumption.[24]

Anthropometrics and Physical Activity

In a meta-analysis of cohort studies, body mass index (BMI), abdominal fatness, and recreational physical activity were not associated with risk of FL, whereas height was positively associated with risk in women (RR = 1.22 for highest vs lowest quartile; 95% CI, 1.01–1.48).[63] In the InterLymph Subtypes Project, FL was not associated with usual adult BMI, but was positively associated with BMI as a young adult (OR = 1.21 per 5 kg/m^2; 95% CI, 1.09–1.35).[24] There was also an association with height (OR = 1.15 for highest vs lowest quartile; 95% CI, 1.02–1.30) restricted to men and no association with physical activity for either sex. The BMI association did not seem to be confounded by other FL risk factors, and similar associations have been observed in the 2 largest cohort studies published to date.[64,65]

Diet

Knowledge of dietary associations with FL has been limited by reliance on case-control studies (with attendant potential biases) and few prospective cohort studies with subtype data or sufficient numbers of FL cases.[4] The most mature results are from a meta-analysis of case-control and cohort studies, which found that vegetable (OR = 0.70 for high vs low intake; 95% CI, 0.53–0.92) but not fruit (OR = 0.96; 95% CI, 0.72–1.28) intake was associated with FL.[66]

INSIGHTS FROM NON-HODGKIN LYMPHOMA SUBTYPE RISK FACTOR PATTERNS

The InterLymph Subtypes Project, which included a variety of risk factor data on 11 NHL subtypes, formally evaluated whether risk factors vary by NHL subtype as well as whether subtypes cluster based on risk factor profiles.[67] With respect to causal het-erogeneity (ie, whether risk factors vary by NHL subtype), **Table 1** summarizes risk factors that were associated with 1 or more NHL subtypes, and, for those with P<.01, a formal heterogeneity test was conducted. For example, family history of NHL was strongly associated with 1 or more NHL subtypes (P = 1.7×10^{-13}) but there was no evidence for subtype heterogeneity (P = .52) across subtypes: 8 of 11 sub-types showed ORs greater than 1.5 (5 at P<.05), including FL. Based on this analysis,

Table 1
Heterogeneity of risk factor associations for follicular lymphoma in the context of other major non-Hodgkin lymphoma subtypes[a]

Risk Factor	P ASSET[b]	NHL OR (95% CI)[d]	P Homogeneity[c]	FL OR (95% CI)[d]	Other Statistically Significant Subtypes (Direction of OR)
Family history of NHL	1.7×10^{-13}	1.79 (1.51–2.13)	0.52	1.99 (1.55–2.59)	MZL (↑), DLBCL (↑), CLL/SLL (↑), MCL (↑)
B cell-activating autoimmune disease	3.8×10^{-22}	1.96 (1.60–2.40)	9.8×10^{-10}	1.27 (0.90–1.79)	MZL (↑), LPL/WM (↑), DLBCL (↑)
Systemic lupus erythematosus	1.9×10^{-8}	2.83 (1.82–4.41)	0.18	1.81 (0.91–3.59)	MF/SS (↑), PTCL (↑), MZL (↑), LPL/WM (↑), DLBCL (↑)
Sjögren syndrome	6.3×10^{-18}	7.52 (3.68–15.4)	7.3×10^{-9}	3.23 (1.19–8.80)	MZL (↑), LPL/WM (↑), DLBCL (↑)
T cell-activating autoimmune disease	0.0053	1.07 (0.95–1.21)	0.012	0.90 (0.72–1.11)	MF/SS (↑), PTCL (↑)
Celiac disease	5.2×10^{-11}	1.77 (1.05–2.99)	5.1×10^{-8}	1.27 (0.53–3.01)	PTCL (↑), DLBCL (↑)
Systemic sclerosis/scleroderma	0.0051	1.03 (0.41–2.58)	0.065	1.08 (0.23–5.00)	MF/SS (↑), BL (↑), HCL (↑)
Hepatitis C virus (seropositive)	2.3×10^{-8}	1.81 (1.39–2.37)	0.0021	0.57 (0.30–1.10)	MZL (↑), LPL/WM (↑), DLBCL (↑), CLL/SLL (↑)
Allergy	5.9×10^{-8}	0.86 (0.81–0.92)	0.24	0.88 (0.79–0.98)	PTCL (↓), DLBCL (↓), CLL/SLL (↓), MCL (↓)
Hay fever	9.1×10^{-9}	0.82 (0.77–0.88)	0.12	0.82 (0.73–0.91)	PTCL (↓), BL (↓), LPL/WM (↓), DLBCL (↓), MCL (↓)
Blood transfusion (ever)	8.8×10^{-5}	0.83 (0.77–0.91)	0.050	0.78 (0.68–0.89)	DLBCL (↓), CLL/SLL (↓), HCL (↓)
Young adult body mass[d]	4.2×10^{-9}	1.95 (1.51–2.53)	0.28	2.13 (1.44–3.14)	DLBCL (↑)
Height[d]	0.0017	1.20 (1.08–1.32)	0.024	1.20 (1.02–1.40)	BL (↑), DLBCL (↑), CLL/SLL (↑), HCL (↑)
Alcohol consumption (≥1 drink/mo)	8.9×10^{-8}	0.87 (0.81–0.93)	0.062	0.86 (0.77–0.96)	MZL (↓), BL (↓), DLBCL (↓), PTCL (↓)
Smoking (duration)[d]	2.2×10^{-9}	1.06 (0.99–1.14)	3.2×10^{-9}	1.19 (1.06–1.33)	PTCL (↑), MZL (↑), LPL/WM (↑), CLL/SLL (↓),

Recreational sun exposure[d]	2.7×10^{-9}	0.74 (0.66–0.83)	0.79	0.70 (0.58–0.84)	PTCL (↓), MZL (↓), DLBCL (↓), CLL/SLL (↓)
Socioeconomic status[d]	3.4×10^{-5}	0.88 (0.83–0.93)	0.061	0.94 (0.85–1.03)	BL (↓), DLBCL (↓), HCL (↑)
General farm worker	0.0082	1.28 (1.10–1.50)	0.34	1.18 (0.88–1.57)	MF/SS (↑), CLL/SLL (↑)
Painter	0.0048	1.22 (0.99–1.51)	0.085	1.31 (0.93–1.84)	MF/SS (↑)
Teacher	5.6×10^{-4}	0.86 (0.77–0.95)	0.0062	0.92 (0.79–1.07)	MZL (↓), BL (↓), DLBCL (↓)

Abbreviations: BL, Burkitt lymphoma; HCL, hairy cell leukemia; LPL, lymphoplasmacytic lymphoma; MF, mycosis fungoides; PTCL, peripheral T-cell lymphoma; SS, Sezary syndrome; WM, Waldenström macroglobulinemia.

[a] Includes the following NHL subtypes: DLBCL; Burkitt lymphoma; peripheral T-cell lymphoma; MZL; CLL/SLL; FL; MCL; lymphoplasmacytic lymphoma/Waldenström macroglobulinemia; mycosis fungoides/Sezary syndrome; hairy cell leukemia.

[b] *P* ASSET is a subset-based statistical approach used to test whether an exposure was associated with 1 or more NHL subtypes.

[c] *P* homogeneity is a test of homogeneity of ORs across NHL subtypes and is derived from the random effects meta-analysis Q statistic.

[d] OR and 95% CI derived from fixed effects logistic regression, adjusted for age, race/ethnicity, sex, and study. OR represents risk per ordinal increase in the following categories: BMI as a young adult (<18.5, 18.5–22.4, 22.5–24.9, 25.0–29.9, ≥30 kg/m²), height (sex-specific quartiles: men, <172.0, 172.0–177.7, 177.8–181.9, ≥182.0 cm; women, <159.0, 159.0–162.9, 163.0–167.9, ≥168.0 cm), duration of cigarette smoking (0, 1–19, 20–29, 30–39, ≥40 years), recreational sun exposure (hours per week, study-specific quartiles), and socioeconomic status (low, medium, high; measured by years of education for studies in North America or by dividing measures of education or socioeconomic status into tertiles for studies in Europe or Australia).

Data from Morton LM, Slager SL, Cerhan JR, et al: Etiologic heterogeneity among non-Hodgkin lymphoma subtypes: the InterLymph Non-Hodgkin Lymphoma Subtypes Project. J Natl Cancer Inst Monogr 2014:130-44, 2014.

there was evidence for subtype heterogeneity of associations ($P<.05$) for most auto-immune diseases, HCV, height, smoking, and occupation as a teacher (FL associations shown in the table). In contrast, homogeneous risks across most subtypes were observed for family history of NHL, allergy/hay fever, blood transfusion, young adult BMI, alcohol use, recreational sun exposure, socioeconomic status, and selected occupations, for which FL showed associations similar to NHL overall and to many other NHL subtypes.

To identify whether certain subtypes shared risk factor profiles, hierarchical clustering was used based on an analysis of all risk factor data simultaneously. Key findings were that B-cell versus T-cell lymphomas first divided into 2 clusters based on risk factor profiles, and then for B-cell lymphomas, MZL, and Burkitt lymphoma formed a cluster, followed by an FL and MCL cluster, a lymphoplasmacytic lymphoma/Waldenström macroglobulinemia and DLBCL cluster, and eventually a CLL/SLL cluster. Overall, no FL-specific risk factors were identified, and, with the exception of autoimmune diseases and HCV, FL largely had a similar risk factor profile that paralleled NHL overall, and most closely matched the risk factor profile for MCL.

OPPORTUNITIES FOR PREVENTION

The descriptive epidemiology of FL, which shows strong international variation and the highest incidence in Western countries, suggests the potential for prevention. The most robust risk factors, including family history, selected autoimmune diseases, and allergy/atopy, provide biological insights but no current direct routes to primary prevention. Definitive genetic loci have been identified but they are limited and not yet sufficiently robust for screening in families or the population. Although there are suggestive leads for modifiable lifestyle and behavioral risk factors that lend themselves to public health interventions (eg, reducing hair dye use, young adult BMI, and smoking), other FL risk factors present more complicated prevention approaches (eg, protective effects of recreational sun exposure and moderate alcohol use), and none of these risk factors are sufficiently established to support interventions. New leads related to certain infections, precursor conditions, and immune biomarkers with FL risk may provide future routes to prevention.

SUMMARY AND FUTURE DIRECTIONS

Progress on identifying FL-specific risk factors has accelerated with the implementation of the InterLymph nested classification as well as with the availability of large pooled analyses. However, beyond family history of NHL, genetic loci, and Sjögren syndrome, there are no established risk factors for FL, although there are promising leads related to atopy, certain infections, hair dye, recreational sun exposure, smoking, alcohol use, and anthropometrics, but these require further research, including better exposure assessment and stronger study designs. Investigators remain early in their understanding of genetic susceptibility to FL, and there are likely to be additional loci identified by GWAS and next-generation sequencing. Deeper understanding of the striking role that HLA plays in FL risk through antigen processing and presentation is needed. Progress on all of these fronts will also allow more robust evaluation of gene-environment interactions. Advances in the understanding of FL biology, through study of both precursors and the genomic and epigenomic architecture of the FL tumor genome, should also help identify novel links to specific risk factors. In addition, most studies have been conducted in Western populations of European ancestry, and future studies need to address racial/ethnic differences and populations of contrasting risk.

DISCLOSURE

The author received NIH grants (R01 CA92153, R01 CA200703, U01 CA195568, and P50 CA97274).

REFERENCES

1. Jaffe ES, Harris NL, Stein H, et al. World Health Organization classification of tumours: pathology and genetics of tumours of haematopoietic and lymphoid tissues. Lyon (France): IARC Press; 2001.
2. Morton LM, Turner JJ, Cerhan JR, et al. Proposed classification of lymphoid neoplasms for epidemiologic research from the Pathology Working Group of the International Lymphoma Epidemiology Consortium (InterLymph). Blood 2007;110: 695–708.
3. Laurent C, Baron M, Amara N, et al. Impact of expert pathologic review of lymphoma diagnosis: study of patients from the French Lymphopath Network. J Clin Oncol 2017;35:2008–17.
4. Cerhan JR, Vajdic CM, Spinelli JJ. The Non-Hodgkin lymphomas. In: Thun MJ, Linet MS, Cerhan JR, et al, editors. Schottenfeld and Fraumeni cancer epidemiology and prevention. 4th edition. New York: Oxford University Press; 2018. p. 767–96.
5. Teras LR, DeSantis CE, Cerhan JR, et al. 2016 US lymphoid malignancy statistics by World Health Organization subtypes. CA Cancer J Clin 2016;66:443–59.
6. Morton LM, Wang SS, Devesa SS, et al. Lymphoma incidence patterns by WHO subtype in the United States, 1992-2001. Blood 2006;107:265–76.
7. Surveillance, Epidemiology, and End Results (SEER) Program (www.seer.cancer. gov) SEER*Stat database: incidence - SEER 18 Regs Research Data + Hurricane Katrina Impacted, Louisiana Cases, Nov 2018 Sub (2000-2016) <Katrina/Rita Population Adjustment> - Linked To County Attributes - Total U.S., 1969-2017 Counties, National Cancer Institute, DCCPS, Surveillance Research Program, released April 2019, based on the November 2018 submission.
8. Perry AM, Diebold J, Nathwani BN, et al. Non-Hodgkin lymphoma in the developing world: review of 4539 cases from the International Non-Hodgkin Lymphoma Classification Project. Haematologica 2016;101:1244–50.
9. van Leeuwen MT, Turner JJ, Joske DJ, et al. Lymphoid neoplasm incidence by WHO subtype in Australia 1982-2006. Int J Cancer 2014;135:2146–56.
10. Sant M, Allemani C, Tereanu C, et al. Incidence of hematologic malignancies in Europe by morphologic subtype: results of the HAEMACARE project. Blood 2010;116:3724–34.
11. Smith A, Crouch S, Lax S, et al. Lymphoma incidence, survival and prevalence 2004-2014: sub-type analyses from the UK's Haematological Malignancy Research Network. Br J Cancer 2015;112:1575–84.
12. Lim RB, Loy EY, Lim GH, et al. Gender and ethnic differences in incidence and survival of lymphoid neoplasm subtypes in an Asian population: secular trends of a population-based cancer registry from 1998 to 2012. Int J Cancer 2015; 137:2674–87.
13. Chihara D, Ito H, Matsuda T, et al. Differences in incidence and trends of haematological malignancies in Japan and the United States. Br J Haematol 2014;164: 536–45.
14. Shirley MH, Sayeed S, Barnes I, et al. Incidence of haematological malignancies by ethnic group in England, 2001-7. Br J Haematol 2013;163:465–77.

15. Dandoit M, Mounier M, Guy J, et al. The heterogeneity of changes in incidence and survival among lymphoid malignancies in a 30-year French population-based registry. Leuk Lymphoma 2015;56:1050–7.

16. Au WY, Gascoyne RD, Klasa RD, et al. Incidence and spectrum of non-Hodgkin lymphoma in Chinese migrants to British Columbia. Br J Haematol 2005;128: 792–6.

17. Sant M, Minicozzi P, Mounier M, et al. Survival for haematological malignancies in Europe between 1997 and 2008 by region and age: results of EUROCARE-5, a population-based study. Lancet Oncol 2014;15:931–42.

18. Nabhan C, Aschebrook-Kilfoy B, Chiu BC, et al. The impact of race, age, and sex in follicular lymphoma: a comprehensive SEER analysis across consecutive treatment eras. Am J Hematol 2014;89:633–8.

19. Junlen HR, Peterson S, Kimby E, et al. Follicular lymphoma in Sweden: nationwide improved survival in the rituximab era, particularly in elderly women: a Swedish Lymphoma Registry study. Leukemia 2015;29:668–76.

20. Maurer MJ, Bachy E, Ghesquieres H, et al. Early event status informs subsequent outcome in newly diagnosed follicular lymphoma. Am J Hematol 2016;91: 1096–101.

21. Sarkozy C, Maurer MJ, Link BK, et al. Cause of death in follicular lymphoma in the first decade of the rituximab era: a pooled analysis of French and US cohorts. J Clin Oncol 2019;37:144–52.

22. Howlader N, Morton LM, Feuer EJ, et al. Contributions of subtypes of non-Hodgkin lymphoma to mortality trends. Cancer Epidemiol Biomarkers Prev 2016;25:174–9.

23. Roulland S, Kelly RS, Morgado E, et al. t(14;18) translocation: a predictive blood biomarker for follicular lymphoma. J Clin Oncol 2014;32:1347–55.

24. Linet MS, Vajdic CM, Morton LM, et al. Medical history, lifestyle, family history, and occupational risk factors for follicular lymphoma: the InterLymph Non-Hodgkin Lymphoma Subtypes Project. J Natl Cancer Inst Monogr 2014;2014:26–40.

25. Fallah M, Kharazmi E, Pukkala E, et al. Familial risk of non-Hodgkin lymphoma by sex, relationship, age at diagnosis and histology: a joint study from five Nordic countries. Leukemia 2016;30:373–8.

26. Goldin LR, Bjorkholm M, Kristinsson SY, et al. Elevated risk of chronic lymphocytic leukemia and other indolent non-Hodgkin's lymphomas among relatives of patients with chronic lymphocytic leukemia. Haematologica 2009;94:647–53.

27. Cerhan JR, Slager SL. Familial predisposition and genetic risk factors for lymphoma. Blood 2015;126:2265–73.

28. Cerhan JR, Braggio E, Slager SL, et al. Genetics in lymphomagenesis. In: Wiernik PH, Dutcher JP, Gertz MA, editors. Neoplastic diseases of the blood. 6th edition. New York: Springer; 2018. p. 723–53.

29. Cerhan JR. Host genetics in follicular lymphoma. Best Pract Res Clin Haematol 2011;24:121–34.

30. Skibola CF, Berndt SI, Vijai J, et al. Genome-wide association study identifies five susceptibility loci for follicular lymphoma outside the HLA region. Am J Hum Genet 2014;95:462–71.

31. List of classifications, agents classified by the IARC monographs. In: IARC monographs on the evaluation of risk to humans, vol. 1-124. IARC; 2019. Retrieved November 7, 2019. Available at: https://monographs.iarc.fr/agents-classified-by-the-iarc/.

32. Dal Maso L, Franceschi S. Hepatitis C virus and risk of lymphoma and other lymphoid neoplasms: a meta-analysis of epidemiologic studies. Cancer Epidemiol Biomarkers Prev 2006;15:2078–85.

33. Anderson LA, Pfeiffer R, Warren JL, et al. Hematopoietic malignancies associated with viral and alcoholic hepatitis. Cancer Epidemiol Biomarkers Prev 2008;17: 3069–75.

34. de Sanjose S, Benavente Y, Vajdic CM, et al. Hepatitis C and non-Hodgkin lymphoma among 4784 cases and 6269 controls from the International Lymphoma Epidemiology Consortium. Clin Gastroenterol Hepatol 2008;6:451–8.

35. Maciocia N, O'Brien A, Ardeshna K. Remission of follicular lymphoma after treatment for Hepatitis C virus infection. N Engl J Med 2016;375:1699–701.

36. Bouvard V, Baan R, Straif K, et al. A review of human carcinogens–Part B: biological agents. Lancet Oncol 2009;10:321–2.

37. Dalia S, Chavez J, Castillo JJ, et al. Hepatitis B infection increases the risk of non-Hodgkin lymphoma: a meta-analysis of observational studies. Leuk Res 2013;37: 1107–15.

38. Clarke CA, Morton LM, Lynch C, et al. Risk of lymphoma subtypes after solid organ transplantation in the United States. Br J Cancer 2013;109:280–8.

39. Ekstrom Smedby K, Vajdic CM, Falster M, et al. Autoimmune disorders and risk of non-Hodgkin lymphoma subtypes: a pooled analysis within the InterLymph Consortium. Blood 2008;111:4029–38.

40. Anderson LA, Gadalla S, Morton LM, et al. Population-based study of autoimmune conditions and the risk of specific lymphoid malignancies. Int J Cancer 2009;125:398–405.

41. Erber E, Lim U, Maskarinec G, et al. Common immune-related risk factors and incident non-Hodgkin lymphoma: the multiethnic cohort. Int J Cancer 2009;125: 1440–5.

42. Hosnijeh FS, Portengen L, Spath F, et al. Soluble B-cell activation marker of sCD27 and sCD30 and future risk of B-cell lymphomas: a nested case-control study and meta-analyses. Int J Cancer 2016;138:2357–67.

43. Kane EV, Roman E, Becker N, et al. Menstrual and reproductive factors, and hormonal contraception use: associations with non-Hodgkin lymphoma in a pooled analysis of InterLymph case-control studies. Ann Oncol 2012;23:2362–74.

44. Kane EV, Bernstein L, Bracci PM, et al. Postmenopausal hormone therapy and non-Hodgkin lymphoma: a pooled analysis of InterLymph case-control studies. Ann Oncol 2013;24:433–41.

45. Kato I, Chlebowski RT, Hou L, et al. Menopausal estrogen therapy and non-Hodgkin's lymphoma: a *post-hoc* analysis of women's health initiative randomized clinical trial. Int J Cancer 2016;138:604–11.

46. Castillo JJ, Mull N, Reagan JL, et al. Increased incidence of non-Hodgkin lymphoma, leukemia, and myeloma in patients with diabetes mellitus type 2: a meta-analysis of observational studies. Blood 2012;119:4845–50.

47. Krishnan B, Morgan GJ. Non-Hodgkin lymphoma secondary to cancer chemotherapy. Cancer Epidemiol Biomarkers Prev 2007;16:377–80.

48. Kim CJ, Freedman DM, Curtis RE, et al. Risk of non-Hodgkin lymphoma after radiotherapy for solid cancers. Leuk Lymphoma 2013;54:1691–7.

49. Castillo JJ, Dalia S, Pascual SK. Association between red blood cell transfusions and development of non-Hodgkin lymphoma: a meta-analysis of observational studies. Blood 2010;116:2897–907.

50. Cerhan JR, Kane E, Vajdic CM, et al. Blood transfusion history and risk of non-Hodgkin lymphoma: an InterLymph pooled analysis. Cancer Causes Control 2019;30:889–900.
51. t Mannetje A, De Roos AJ, Boffetta P, et al. Occupation and risk of non-hodgkin lymphoma and its subtypes: a pooled analysis from the InterLymph consortium. Environ Health Perspect 2016;124:396–405.
52. Koutros S, Harris SA, Spinelli JJ, et al. Non-Hodgkin lymphoma risk and organo-phosphate and carbamate insecticide use in the North American pooled project. Environ Int 2019;127:199–205.
53. Schinasi L, Leon ME. Non-Hodgkin lymphoma and occupational exposure to agricultural pesticide chemical groups and active ingredients: a systematic review and meta-analysis. Int J Environ Res Public Health 2014;11:4449–527.
54. Leon ME, Schinasi LH, Lebailly P, et al. Pesticide use and risk of non-Hodgkin lymphoid malignancies in agricultural cohorts from France, Norway and the USA: a pooled analysis from the AGRICOH consortium. Int J Epidemiol 2019;48:1519–35.
55. Zhang Y, Sanjose SD, Bracci PM, et al. Personal use of hair dye and the risk of certain subtypes of non-Hodgkin lymphoma. Am J Epidemiol 2008;167:1321–31.
56. Kricker A, Armstrong BK, Hughes AM, et al. Personal sun exposure and risk of non Hodgkin lymphoma: a pooled analysis from the Interlymph Consortium. Int J Cancer 2008;122:144–54.
57. Park HY, Hong YC, Lee K, et al. Vitamin D status and risk of non-Hodgkin lymphoma: an updated meta-analysis. PLoS One 2019;14:e0216284.
58. Castillo JJ, Dalia S. Cigarette smoking is associated with a small increase in the incidence of non-Hodgkin lymphoma: a meta-analysis of 24 observational studies. Leuk Lymphoma 2012;53:1911–9.
59. Sergentanis TN, Kanavidis P, Michelakos T, et al. Cigarette smoking and risk of lymphoma in adults: a comprehensive meta-analysis on Hodgkin and non-Hodgkin disease. Eur J Cancer Prev 2013;22:131–50.
60. Diver WR, Patel AV, Thun MJ, et al. The association between cigarette smoking and non-Hodgkin lymphoid neoplasms in a large US cohort study. Cancer Causes Control 2012;23:1231–40.
61. Tramacere I, Pelucchi C, Bonifazi M, et al. Alcohol drinking and non-Hodgkin lymphoma risk: a systematic review and a meta-analysis. Ann Oncol 2012;23:2791–8.
62. Psaltopoulou T, Sergentanis TN, Ntanasis-Stathopoulos I, et al. Alcohol consumption and risk of hematological malignancies: a meta-analysis of prospective studies. Int J Cancer 2018;143:486–95.
63. Psaltopoulou T, Sergentanis TN, Ntanasis-Stathopoulos I, et al. Anthropometric characteristics, physical activity and risk of hematological malignancies: a systematic review and meta-analysis of cohort studies. Int J Cancer 2019;145:347–59.
64. Bertrand KA, Giovannucci E, Zhang SM, et al. A prospective analysis of body size during childhood, adolescence, and adulthood and risk of non-Hodgkin lymphoma. Cancer Prev Res (Phila) 2013;6:864–73.
65. Yang TO, Cairns BJ, Kroll ME, et al. Body size in early life and risk of lymphoid malignancies and histological subtypes in adulthood. Int J Cancer 2016;139:42–9.
66. Chen GC, Lv DB, Pang Z, et al. Fruits and vegetables consumption and risk of non-Hodgkin's lymphoma: a meta-analysis of observational studies. Int J Cancer 2013;133:190–200.
67. Morton LM, Slager SL, Cerhan JR, et al. Etiologic heterogeneity among non-Hodgkin lymphoma subtypes: the InterLymph Non-Hodgkin Lymphoma Subtypes Project. J Natl Cancer Inst Monogr 2014;2014:130–44.

Clinical and Biological Prognostic Factors in Follicular Lymphoma

Anand A. Patel, MD[a], Sonali M. Smith, MD[b],*

KEYWORDS

- Follicular lymphoma • Biological risk factors • Clinical risk factors
- Prognostic indices

KEY POINTS

- Current prognostic factors span both clinical and biological data. They aid in risk stratification but do not play in role in starting treatment.
- Prognostic factors at diagnosis of follicular lymphoma include histology, genetic aberrations, tumor microenvironment, prognostic indices, and tumor burden.
- Salient prognostic factors over the course of treatment include PET status at the end of induction treatment, progression of disease within 24 months, CR at 30 months, and double-refractory disease.
- Prognostic factors with emerging relevance include measurable residual disease and vitamin D.
- Future prognostic tools will need to synchronize both clinical and biological data to augment individual-level decision making.

INTRODUCTION

Approximately 75,000 people are diagnosed with non-Hodgkin lymphoma on a yearly basis, with follicular lymphoma (FL) comprising of 20% to 30% of these cases and representing 70% of all indolent lymphoma cases.[1–3] The median survival in the modern era has steadily improved and now approaches several decades for the majority of patients. However, FL is quite heterogeneous and mortality from either lymphoma progression or treatment-related complications remains problematic. Most patients are subjected to repeated courses of therapy interspersed with periods of observation.[4] Given the broad range of clinical outcomes in FL, prognostic factors are highly

a Department of Medicine, Section of Hematology-Oncology, University of Chicago, 5841 South Maryland Avenue, Room E-212A, MC2115, Chicago, IL 60637, USA; b Section of Hematology/Oncology, Lymphoma Program, Department of Medicine, The University of Chicago, 5841 South Maryland Avenue, MC2115, Chicago, IL 60637, USA
* Corresponding author.
E-mail address: smsmith@medicine.bsd.uchicago.edu
Twitter: @Anand_88_Patel (A.A.P.); @SoniSmithMD (S.M.S.)

Hematol Oncol Clin N Am 34 (2020) 647–662
https://doi.org/10.1016/j.hoc.2020.02.002
0889-8588/20/© 2020 Elsevier Inc. All rights reserved.

valuable in helping to identify high-risk populations at risk of inferior outcomes. Although early identification of the highest risk patients is quite difficult at an individual level, prognostic factors both at the time of diagnosis and ones that become available over the course of treatment provide valuable insight into predicted outcomes for patients with FL.

In the current age of FL, prognostic factors at diagnosis include pathologic data, genetic aberrations of the disease, the tumor microenvironment (TME), clinical indices, and tumor burden. In addition, high-risk disease can become apparent during the course of treatment by evaluating the response to therapy and the duration of response. Unfortunately, these factors aid in risk stratification but do not play a role in determining when to start treatment or which treatment option to implement. In this review, we aimed to summarize the current prognostic factors available to clinicians caring for patients with FL while also commenting on emerging prognostic factors.

PROGNOSTIC FACTORS AT INITIAL DIAGNOSIS
Histologic Grade

Histologic grade is one of the earliest approaches to determining disease behavior. The World Health Organization classification of histologic grade in FL is divided into grades 1, 2, 3A, and 3B; 3A is classified by the presence of centrocytes and 3B is classified by sheets of centroblasts despite preservation of the follicular structure.[5] Grade 1 and grade 2 FL can be difficult to distinguish from each other, and the most recent World Health Organization classification lumps these together as FL1-2 (also called FL, low grade). FL1-2 typically behaves in an indolent fashion. The prognostic implication of grade 3A (FL3a) has been more controversial, with some practitioners treating similarly to FL1-2 and others considering this to be a more aggressive entity. Most will agree that grade 3b FL (FL3b) is akin to diffuse large B-cell lymphoma (DLBCL) based on cytogenetics, immunohistochemistry, and gene expression analysis.[6,7]

Previous studies have reported conflicting data regarding the prognostic implication of FL3a. Wahlin and colleagues[8] evaluated a very heterogeneously treated FL population and found a similar median overall survival between FL1-2 and FL3 patients. The prognostic role of histologic grade in a cohort of patients treated with rituximab-based regimens without chemotherapy was studied as well. Patients with FL3a disease were found to have a 6-year freedom from time to next treatment rate of 62% in comparison with 39% for FL2 patients and 22% for FL1 patients.[9] A recent analysis of the Southwest Oncology Group (SWOG) S0016 prospective phase III clinical trial cohort sought to assess the prognostic impact of histologic grade on a chemoimmunotherapy-treated FL population. There were 491 patients analyzed, with 452 cases being classified as FL1-2 and 39 with FL3a. Only 1 patient was found to have FL3b disease and was not included in analysis. The 10-year overall survival was 79% in the FL1-2 group and 68% in the FL3a group, but this numerical difference did not meet statistical significance. The 10-year progression-free survival was 49% in the FL1-2 group and 47% in the FL3a group.[10] Of note, all 3 studies required pathology review of specimens owing to previously reported high inter-rater variability in assigning grade.[8–10] Given the variability in assigning histologic grade, as well as the potential impact of treatment delivered, it may be an inconsistent means of determining prognosis in patients with newly diagnosed FL.

Cytogenetics

FL frequently has both cytogenetic and molecular aberrations, and their prognostic usefulness is emerging. The t(14;18) translocation is a genetic hallmark of FL, resulting in juxtaposition of *BCL2* with *IGH*, thereby causing increased expression of the antia-poptotic BCL2 protein. Although *t(14;18)* is considered an initial event in FL pathogen-esis and is present in approximately 85% of patients, it can be found in healthy individuals as well. Summers and colleagues[11] found that 23% of healthy individuals have detectable *BCL2/IGH* rearrangement. Later studies reported that healthy individuals with a *t(14;18)* frequency of 1 in 10,000 blood cells had a 23-fold greater risk of progressing to FL.[12] Thus, *t(14;18)* seems to be an initial and perhaps a requisite event, although the majority of people with the rearrangement do not develop FL. Approximately 10% of patients with FL do not have *t(14;18)* and although the gene expression profile (GEP) of this subset differs significantly from *t(14;18)*-positive patients, there does not seem to be prognostic significance associated with *t(14;18)*.[13,14]

In addition to *t(14;18)*, there are a number of other recurrent chromosomal aberrations noted in FL. Studies from the prerituximab era have noted inferior prognosis associated with deletion of 6q and deletion of 17p.[5,15,16] A more recent analysis of chromosomal aberrations detected by G-banding was carried out by Mitsui and colleagues.[17] Two hundred one samples from patients with FL were analyzed and 87.1% of them had rituximab-based therapy. The initial analysis revealed deletion 17p, abnormalities in chromosome 3q27, trisomy 7, trisomy 21, or a complex karyotype (≥3 chromosomal aberrations) as having inferior overall survival. Upon conducting multivariate analysis, however, only trisomy 21 was identified as having prognostic significance. Patients with trisomy 21 had a 3-year progression-free survival of 27.8% and a 3-year overall survival of 45.5% compared with 64.2% and 96.1%, respectively, in patients without trisomy 21. Of note, very few patients harbor trisomy 21, limiting broader applicability.

Evaluation of chromosomal abnormalities within the SWOG S0016 cohort using chromosome genomic array testing has also been reported. Early progression was correlated with 2p gain and 2p loss of heterozygosity. A 9p deletion, where *CDKN2A/B* are housed, correlated with worse progression-free survival. A 16p deletion, where *CREBBP* is housed, and a 17p deletion were both prognostic for poorer overall survival.[18] The routine use of chromosome genomic array testing in patients with FL may allow for more accurate risk stratification as it better identifies cytogenetic abnormalities in comparison with fluorescence in situ hybridization, but this tool is reserved for research settings at the moment.

Genetic Mutations

Over the last decade, the genetic landscape of FL has been better elucidated via next-generation sequencing assays. A wide variety of chromatin-modifying gene mutations have been identified in FL, with the most common ones being *KMT2D* (approximately 75%), *CREBBP* (approximately 65%), and *EZH2* (approximately 25%).[19–21] These mutations are primarily involved in histone modification. Although the presence of chromatin-modifying genetic mutations are thought to be essential to the pathogenesis of FL, specific genetic mutations do not seem to have prognostic implications. The M7-FLIPI prognostic score incorporates epigenetic gene mutations in *EZH2*, *CREBBP*, *ARID1A*, *MEF2B*, and *EP300*.[22] The 2 additional gene mutations used in the M7-FLIPI are *FOXO1* and *CARD11*. *FOXO1* is a transcription factor essential to cell survival and proliferation and *CARD11* is involved in lymphocyte activation. Both mutations are seen more frequently in FL that has transformed into DLBCL.[23,24]

Genetic aberrations in 2 tumor suppressor genes have been shown to have independent prognostic implications: *TP53* and *CDK2NA*. Mutations in the tumor suppressor gene *TP53* are found in 6% of previously untreated FL cases. The presence of a *TP53* mutation predicts for inferior progression-free survival and overall survival even when controlling for the International Prognostic Index (IPI).[25] In addition, acquisition of *TP53* mutations has been found in 28% of patients with FL that transform into DLBCL.[26] Deletion or methylation of *CDK2NA* was found in 27% of pretreatment FL samples. The presence of either *CDK2NA* aberration was associated with poorer overall survival, particularly in patients treated with rituximab.[27]

Kridel and colleagues[28] evaluated clonal populations in FL samples taken at the time of transformation or progression of disease. Their findings highlight differences in the genetic mutations associated with early progression in comparison to those seen in transformation. Genetic mutations implicated in early progression include *KMT2C*, *BTG1*, *TP53*, *MKI67*, *XBP1*, *SOCS1*, *IKZF3*, *B2M*, *FAS*, and *MYD88*. Genetic mutations implicated in transformation were *TP53*, *B2M*, *EZH2*, *MYC*, *CCND3*, *EBF1*, *PIM1*, *GNA13*, *ITPKB*, *CHD8*, *P2RY8*, and *S1PR2*. Correia and colleagues[29] separately studied the role of *BCL2* mutations on prognostic outcomes and found a higher risk of transformation and shorter overall survival. In summary, although the genetic landscape in FL has become better defined, continued evaluation of recurrent abnormalities will be necessary to determine their role in prognosis.

Tumor Microenvironment

In addition to the molecular aberrations found with tumor cells, the composition of the TME of FL has prognostic significance as well. Dave and colleagues[30] first highlighted the potential importance of the TME of FL with regards to prognosis. Using a GEP of the nonmalignant immune cells present in biopsy specimens, they were able to identify 2 signatures termed as immune response 1 (IR1) and immune response 2 (IR2). IR1 included T-cell–restricted genes, along with genes more highly expressed in monocytes, whereas IR2 included genes highly expressed in monocytes, dendritic cells, or both types of cells. IR1 was associated with a better overall survival, but its roles in applicability are unclear. Limitations of this analysis include the lack of clinical availability, inconsistent reproducibility of these results, and no widely available surrogate markers to characterize an IR1 or IR2 signature. However, characterizing the prognostic role of the TME in FL continues to be of great interest.[31] The presence of programmed death-1–expressing cells is associated with improved overall survival, whereas a decrease in these cells is observed in transformation.[32,33] A 23-gene panel meant to reflect both B-cell biology and TME was recently studied in the PRIMA clinical trial cohort, all of which received chemoimmunotherapy. This gene panel was selected from 395 genes correlated with a risk of progression to build a predictive model. A low-risk and high-risk predictor score were identified; a high-risk GEP score was associated with inferior progression-free survival and progression of disease within 24 months (POD24); this was validated in 3 separate cohorts.[34] The high-risk GEP score was also found to correlate highly with the ICA13 gene signature, which is enriched in germinal center centroblasts and Burkitt lymphoma. Of note, both the IR1 and IR2 gene signature described by Dave and colleagues were not predictive of progression-free survival in the Huet cohort, perhaps reflecting that the Dave cohort was rituximab naive.[30,34] In addition, the 23-gene panel was primarily evaluated in a high tumor burden population and further studies will be necessary to validate its use in the low-tumor burden FL population. It remains to be seen whether the 23-gene GEP score can be used to guide treatment decisions by identification of low-risk populations, and validation in other datasets is ongoing.

Clinical Prognostic Indices

Clinical prognostic indices have the advantage of being easily available with basic clinical and laboratory assessments. The IPI, combining 5 readily available factors, was derived by analysis of the aggressive non-Hodgkin lymphoma population and is predictive of progression-free survival and overall survival.[35] When applied to the FL population, however, the IPI provides little prognostic discrimination between lower risk and intermediate risk groups; in addition, only 11.2% of patients with FL were in the high risk group, thus limiting its broader applicability.[36]

The Follicular Lymphoma IPI (FLIPI), designed to be more specific for this population, was derived by retrospective analysis of 4167 patients diagnosed between 1985 and 1992 and powered to predict overall survival. A multivariate analysis identified 5 prognostic features, including age greater than 60 years, Ann Arbor Stage III/IV, hemoglobin less than 12 g/dL, 4 or more nodal areas, and increased lactate dehydrogenase (**Table 1**). Patients were classified as low risk (5-year overall survival of 90.6%, 10-year overall survival of 70.7%), intermediate risk (5-year overall survival of 77.6%, 10-year overall survival of 50.9%), and high risk (5-year overall survival of 52.5%, 10-year overall survival of 35.5%).[37] Initial criticism of the FLIPI included its derivation from a prerituximab era; however, the FLIPI has subsequently been validated as a robust tool in rituximab-treated patient cohorts as well.[38–40] The FLIPI2 was developed from 942 patients with FL treated in a more modern era, although only 59% of patients received a rituximab-containing regimen. All data had been collected prospectively and allowed for analysis of variables that were incomplete in the FLIPI cohort, including beta-2-microglobulin. The FLIPI2 score is composed of age greater than 60 year old, elevated beta-2-microglobulin, bone marrow involvement, diameter of an involved lymph node greater than 6 cm, and hemoglobin less than 12 g/dL level (see **Table 1**). In contrast with the original FLIPI, the FLIPI2 was designed with progression-free survival as the primary end point. Three groups with distinct outcomes were identified, with 3-year progression-free survival as 91%, 69%, and 51% in the low-, intermediate-, and high-risk groups, respectively. When restricted to rituximab-treated patients, FLIPI2 remained prognostic with 3-year progression-free survival rates of 89%, 73%, and 57% for the low-, intermediate-, and high-risk groups, respectively. Overall survival was analyzed in the entire cohort and met statistical significance, with a 5-year overall survival of 98%, 88%, and 77% for the low-, intermediate-, and high-risk groups, respectively.[41] In practice, the FLIPI continues to be more commonly used owing to validation across multiple large cohorts and because beta-2-microglobulin is not routinely collected in clinical practice. Despite this latter consideration, the French cooperative group performed an analysis on patients with FL uniformly treated with chemoimmunotherapy and identified 2 factors predictive of outcome: bone marrow involvement and serum beta-2-microglobulin. This simplified prognostic index, called the PRIMA-PI, offers prognostic information related to both progression-free survival and overall survival.[40] Although the simplicity of PRIMA-PI is appealing, further validation is necessary for wider incorporation and to change routine clinical practice. In addition, beta-2-microglobulin is not routinely assessed by all practitioners.

Given the burgeoning molecular and genomic data, several groups have collaborated to develop a prognostic tool inclusive of these features. The M7-FLIPI score incorporates both mutational information and clinical parameters to help determine prognosis in patients with FL. Pastore and colleagues[22] performed DNA deep sequencing on 151 FL biopsy specimens collected from patients on GLSG2000, a prospective phase III clinical trial using frontline chemoimmunotherapy. Analysis of 74 genes was performed, with the identification of 7 genes (*EZH2*, *ARID1A*, *MEF2B*, *EP300*, *FOXO1*, *CREBBP*, and *CARD11*) as holding prognostic significance based on a multivariable risk analysis and the frequency of mutations. Of interest, these mutations were not prognostic by themselves, but nicely enhanced clinical parameters

Table 1
Clinical prognostic indices in FL

Prognostic Index	Prognostic Factors	Outcomes	Notes	Reference
IPI	Performance status Extranodal sites Serum lactate dehydrogenase Ann Arbor stage Age	5-y overall survival: Low risk: 73% Low intermediate risk: 51% High–intermediate risk: 43% High risk: 26%	Developed in aggressive non-Hodgkin lymphoma population Poor discrimination between low-risk and intermediate-risk FL populations	The International Non-Hodgkin's Lymphoma Prognostic Factors Project,[35] 1993
FLIPI	Number of nodal sites Hemoglobin Serum lactate dehydrogenase Ann Arbor stage Age	5-y overall survival: Low risk: 91% Intermediate risk: 78% High risk: 52%	Developed in the prerituximab era Has been validated in rituximab-treated populations	Solal-Céligny et al,[37] 2004
FLIPI2	Hemoglobin Serum beta-2-microglobulin Longest diameter of large involved node Bone marrow involvement Age	5-y overall survival: Low risk: 98% Intermediate risk: 88% High risk: 77%	59% of patients received rituximab Progression-free survival used as a primary end point for the model	Federico et al,[41] 2009
PRIMA-PI	Bone marrow involvement Serum beta-2-microglobulin	5-y overall survival: Low/intermediate risk: 93% High risk: 81%	Progression-free survival used as a primary end point for the model	Bachy et al,[40] 2018
M7-FLIPI	Mutational data (EZH2, ARID1A, MEF2B, EP300, FOXO1, CREBBP, and CARD11) Performance status FLIPI factors	5-y overall survival: Low risk: 90% High risk: 65%	May not hold prognostic significance in patients treated with chemotherapy-free rituximab regimens	Pastore et al,[22] 2015

Data from Refs.[22,35,37,40,41]

including the FLIPI and performance status (see **Table 1**). Specifically, the M7-FLIPI score combines the mutational status in those 7 genes, FLIPI, and performance status. Patients were stratified to low risk or high risk based on M7-FLIPI score; patients with high-risk M7-FLIPI had a 5-year overall survival of 65.25% and 5-year failure-free survival of 38.29% compared with a 5-year overall survival of 89.98% and 5-year failure-free survival 65.25% in the low-risk group. The M7-FLIPI outperformed the FLIPI in a validation cohort and outperformed FLIPI2 in the subset of patients on GLSG2000, where it could be calculated.[22] Of note, a recent analysis of M7-FLIPI in patients treated with chemotherapy-free rituximab regimens failed to find prognostic significance.[42] Further work is necessary to evaluate the usefulness of M7-FLIPI in patients with FL with low tumor burden and those treated with chemotherapy-free rituximab regimens.

It is difficult to determine the true applicability of these prognostic indices in practice. Although the modern era holds a number of prognostic indices of value in large FL populations, to date they have not been helpful in making treatment decisions, particularly at an individual level. Symptomatic disease, as reflected by the Groupe D'Etude des Lymphomes Folliculaires criteria or National Comprehensive Cancer Network guidelines continue to be the most commonly used criteria for initiating treatment in FL.[43,44] A second issue is that the prognostic indices may depend on the patient population tested; both the PRIMA-PI and the M7-FLIPI are likely most relevant in patients with a high tumor burden treated with chemoimmunotherapy. The key usefulness of the prognostic indices may be the ability to compare populations across clinical trials and to provide a general sense of prognosis for individual patients.

Baseline Imaging as a Prognostic Indicator

The use of PET/computed tomography (CT) scans in the initial staging evaluation of FL has become increasingly commonplace and FL is a highly PET-avid disease (**Table 2**). The National Comprehensive Cancer Network guidelines recommend baseline PET/CT scans for more accurate staging and to evaluate for potential areas of transformation.[44] Meignan and colleagues[45] performed a pooled analysis of patients enrolled in 3 prospective studies treated with chemoimmunotherapy. All patients met the criteria for high tumor burden or advanced disease. Baseline PET/CT scans in 185 patients

Table 2 PET scan usefulness in FL		
Time in Treatment Course	Poor Prognostic Risk Factors	Reference
Time of diagnosis	High TMTV Bone marrow involvement Splenic involvement Soft tissue involvement >2 nodal sites	Meignan et al,[45] 2016; St-Pierre et al,[46] 2019
End of induction therapy	PET positivity Lack of complete response by 2007 IHC Lack of complete response by 2014 Lugano criteria	Trotman et al,[48] 2014; Cottereau et al,[49] 2018; Trotman et al,[50] 2018

Abbreviation: IHC, International Harmonization Criteria.
Data from Refs.[45,46,48-50]

were used to calculate the tumor metabolic total volume (TMTV). The median TMTV was 297 cm^3 and a cutoff of 510 cm^3 was determined as the optimal cutoff for progression-free survival and overall survival. Of these patients, 29% were classified as having high TMTV, with a 5-year progression-free survival of 32.7% and a 5-year overall survival of 84.8% compared with 65.1% and 94.7%, respectively, in patients with lower TMTV. Higher TMTV was also significantly associated with stage III/IV disease, extranodal/bone marrow involvement, and higher FLIPI/FLIPI2 scores. TMTV was used in combination with FLIPI2 score to identify 3 prognostic groups: (1) low TMTV plus FLIPI2 score of 0 to 2, (2) high TMTV or FLIPI2 score of 3 to 5, and (3) high TMTV plus FLIPI2 score 3 to 5. The predicted 5-year overall survival was excellent, despite high- or low-risk disease at 99%, 85%, and 87% for groups 1, 2, and 3, respectively, with no significant difference between the latter 2 groups.

The site and extent of disease involvement on baseline PET/CT has been found to have prognostic significance as well. A single-center retrospective review of baseline PET/CT scans in 613 patients with PET/CT imaging found that more than 2 nodal sites, splenic involvement, bony involvement, and soft tissue involvement were all significantly associated with failure to achieve event-free survival at 24 months with multivariate analysis.[46] Although the use of TMTV in prognostic assessment of FL is very promising, the lack of standardization regarding PET/CT scans, existence of multiple methods of calculating TMTV, and variable use of a specific cutoff point to identify a high TMTV population challenge TMTV as a widespread means of initial FL prognostic assessment.[47]

PROGNOSTIC FACTORS DURING THE COURSE OF TREATMENT

As discussed elsewhere in this article, there are a number of challenges to identifying prognosis (particularly at an individual level) at initial diagnosis, likely reflecting significant disease heterogeneity. In contrast, several parameters after initial treatment are emerging as robust prognostic factors. Specifically, response to induction therapy, duration of response, development of double refractoriness, and the identification of measurable residual disease (MRD) are becoming increasingly useful.

End of Induction Imaging

PET/CT scans at the end of induction treatment may be very helpful in further clarifying prognosis in patients with FL (see **Table 2**). Trotman and colleagues[48] conducted a pooled analysis of 3 clinical trial cohorts treated with chemoimmunotherapy. All included patients that had end of induction PET/CT scans within 3 months of induction therapy. Seventeen percent of patients had a positive PET/CT scan at that time; patients with a positive PET/CT scan had lower rates of 4-year progression-free survival (23.2% vs 63.4%), lower median progression-free survival (16.9 months vs 74 months), and 4-year overall survival (87.2% vs 97.1%). Cottereau and colleagues[49] analyzed 159 patients in multicenter prospective studies that had both baseline PET/CT scans and end of induction scans; PET positivity at end of induction predicted inferior 5-year progression-free survival (26.9% vs 59.6) and 5-year overall survival (84.0% vs 93.3%) when compared with PET-negative patients. End of induction imaging was also analyzed in the GALLIUM clinical trial cohort. There were 595 patients who had both baseline PET/CT scans and end of induction PET/CT scans available for analysis.[50] Complete CT response by the 2007 International Harmonization Criteria, complete PET response by the 2007 International Harmonization Criteria, and complete PET response by the 2014 Lugano criteria were all predictive of progression-free survival at 30 months.[50] However, only PET response by the 2007 International Harmonization Criteria and PET response by the 2014 Lugano criteria were predictive for overall survival, suggesting that end of induction response by PET scan may be more useful than CT assessment.

Time to Relapse

Early relapse after induction therapy has been identified as a risk factor for inferior overall survival. An analysis of the National Lymphocare Study was performed and identified 588 patients with FL treated with frontline R-CHOP. Of these patients, 19% achieved POD24. This group was more likely to have higher FLIPI scores compared with patients without early POD. The 5-year overall survival was 50% in patients with early POD compared with 90% in patients without early POD.[51] An analysis of the PRIMA trial cohort also found POD24 to predict inferior overall survival.[40] Both the Lymphocare cohort and the PRIMA cohort had undergone treatment with rituximab in addition to combination chemotherapy. The POD24-PI is a prognostic index designed to identify patients at risk of POD24; it includes FLIPI and genetic mutations in *EP300*, *FOXO1*, and *EZH2*. However, M7-FLIPI was found to be more accurate than POD24-PI at predicting POD24.[52] The PRIMA-PI also has predictive usefulness with regard to POD24.[40]

As more patients with FL receive chemotherapy-free regimens, it will be essential to validate the prognostic usefulness of POD24 in this population. Moccia and colleagues[53] recently reported the validity of POD24 in a cohort treated with chemotherapy-free regimens. In addition, an analysis of 111 patients with FL treated with rituximab monotherapy identified failure to achieve event-free survival at 12 months to be associated with poorer overall survival; this finding needs validation in a larger cohort.[54] With regard to postinduction surveillance, imaging is not routinely done at the 24-month mark and identification of this high-risk population is therefore probably incomplete. An interesting question is whether a 24-month scan should be done to identify additional POD24 patients. Clinical trials to identify the best treatment strategy in the POD24 population are also ongoing; the SWOG Cancer Research Network is currently evaluating the role of obinutuzumab both combined with chemotherapy and in chemotherapy-free regimens (NCT 03269669).

Double-Refractory Disease

Although not consistently defined, it is clear that patients with primary refractory disease or early relapse following either rituximab or alkylating agents have a poor prognosis. Rituximab refractory is typically defined as nonresponse or relapse within 6 months of exposure and has been used to develop therapeutic agents. For example, the GADOLIN study tested bendamustine plus obinutuzumab versus bendamustine in rituximab-refractory indolent lymphomas, leading to approval by the US Food and Drug Administration for this regimen.[55] The concept of double-refractory disease extends this definition to include early relapse (within 6 months) or refractory disease after an alkylator-based regimen, typically bendamustine or cyclophosphamide. Idelalisib, the first PI3Kδ inhibitor approved by the US Food and Drug Administration in indolent lymphomas, was entirely based on assessing efficacy in patients with less than a partial response or disease progression within 6 months after completion of the prior regimen.[56] There is no robust dataset showing the expected specific survival (ie, a baseline), but this is clearly an area of unmet need and poor prognosis where new agents should be pursued.

Duration of Complete Remission

In addition to POD24, sustained complete remissions have prognostic significance. Approximately 3800 patients with FL across 13 randomized controlled trials were analyzed to determine the prognostic significance of CR at 30 months after the initiation of induction therapy. Of note, the trial populations included chemotherapy, immunotherapy, and chemoimmunotherapy-treated patients. An odds ratio of 11.8 was found, meaning there are significantly higher odds of progression-free survival if CR at 30 months is achieved. Secondary analysis of CR at 24 months demonstrated a high correlation with progression-free survival as well; however, a post hoc analysis was used for this end point.[57] Identification of the biologic and clinical factors common to patients with CR at 30 months will be necessary to try and identify these patients at diagnosis or earlier in the course of treatment.

Measurable Residual Disease

Finding means of identifying residual disease at increasingly sensitive levels has become a major area of research across oncology. In the FL population, this has been studied using cell-free DNA and circulating tumor cells. At diagnosis, cell-free DNA and circulating tumor cell burden correlate with TMTV and are independently predictive of progression-free survival.[58] MRD detection during treatment may have prognostic implications as well.

Polymerase chain reaction (PCR)-based methods to detect *BCL2/IGH* rearrangement as a means of tracking MRD have been studied for many years within the FL population. Although previous studies have shown poorer progression-free survival and overall survival with MRD positivity in FL, there has been controversy regarding regular use of MRD status in clinical practice owing to heterogeneity in sample source, assay sensitivity, and change in treatment modalities.[59] Two recent studies have evaluated PCR-based testing of MRD status and its prognostic significance. Zohren and colleagues[60] prospectively evaluated MRD in a phase III clinical trial cohort receiving chemoimmunotherapy. MRD was assessed via PCR on a peripheral blood sample; failure to achieve MRD negativity after treatment was associated with a hazard ratio of 3.15 with regard to progression-free survival. The GALLIUM study, a large international phase III trial comparing obinutuzumab chemotherapy with rituximab chemotherapy, is evaluating MRD data. Preliminary results show that achievement of MRD negativity in both treatment arms is associated with improved progression-free survival.[61] Of note, obinutuzumab-containing regimens are more likely to achieve MRD negativity, although this is only significant in non–bendamustine-containing regimens. Pulsoni and colleagues[62] retrospectively evaluated 42 patients with early stage FL with detectable *BCL2/IGH* rearrangement via PCR of peripheral blood or bone marrow sample at diagnosis. The patients then underwent involved-field radiation therapy with repeat PCR evaluation of *BCR2/IGH* rearrangement. Patients were classified as having undetectable MRD, a tumor burden of less than 1×10^{-5} cells, or a tumor burden of greater than 1×10^{-5}. Patients with MRD negativity had significantly improved progression-free survival; in addition, patients with MRD positivity after involved-field radiation therapy who underwent rituximab consolidation had improved progression-free survival compared with those who did not receive rituximab. Neither study directly evaluated prognostic implications on overall survival. The use of circulating tumor cells as a means of monitoring MRD has not been evaluated in a post-treatment setting.

RISK FACTORS FOR TRANSFORMATION

Transformation of FL to DLBCL has typically portended poorer overall survival and, therefore, an analysis of risk factors at initial presentation and during the course of treatment that predict for transformation are of great clinical interest.[63,64] Wagner-

Johnston and colleagues[65] reported on clinical risk factors predictive for transformation in the National Lymphocare Study cohort; these included ECOG performance status of greater than 1, involvement of more than 1 extranodal sites, elevated lactate dehydrogenase, and the presence of B-symptoms at diagnosis. The 5-year overall survival in transformed FL patients was 75% compared with 95% in patients with FL without transformation. Multivariate analysis of the PRIMA cohort by Sarkozy and colleagues[66] identified an ECOG performance status or greater than 1 and a hemoglobin of less than 12 g/dL at presentation as independent risk factors for transformation. A number of genetic aberrations are increased in transformed FL including mutations in *FOXO1*, *CARD11*, *TP53*, *B2M*, *EZH2*, *MYC*, *CCND3*, *EBF1*, *PIM1*, *GNA13*, *ITPKB*, *CHD8*, *P2RY8*, *S1PR2*, and *BCL2*.[23,24,26,28,29] Regarding the TME, a decrease in programmed death-1–expressing cells has been associated with transformation.[32,33] In addition to assessable risk factors at diagnosis, POD24 after treatment with chemoimmunotherapy has been reported as a risk factor for transformation as well.[66,67] Treatment itself may also have an impact on risk of transformation; an analysis of 8116 patients with FL identified a 10-year cumulative hazard of transformation of 7.7%, with a significant difference in those treated with rituximab (a 10-year hazard of 5.2%) and those who were not (a 10-year hazard of 8.7%).[68] Although a number of risk factors associated with overall survival also predict for transformation, considerations for the risk of transformation based on initiation of treatment and its subsequent impact on survival needs further exploration.

EMERGING PROGNOSTIC FACTORS

As we continue to refine current prognostic factors available for FL, newer prognostic factors are undergoing investigation as well. Serum vitamin D levels have been studied in relation to clinical outcomes in FL. Kelly and colleagues[69] evaluated the vitamin D levels of patients enrolled in the SWOG S9800, SWOG S9911, SWOG S0016, or LYSA PRIMA clinical trials, all of which incorporated chemoimmunotherapy as treatment. Patients with vitamin D levels of less than 20 ng/mL in the SWOG cohort had statistically increased risk of progression-free survival and overall survival; an association between vitamin D insufficiency and poorer outcome was noted in the LYSA cohort, but statistical significance was not reached. Vitamin D insufficiency in a cohort of Mayo Clinic/University of Iowa patients with FL treated with chemoimmunotherapy was predictive of poorer rates of event-free survival at 12 months, overall survival, and lymphoma-specific survival.[70] However, previous observational studies looking at the

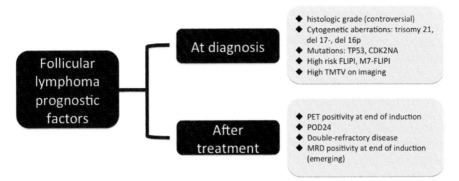

Fig. 1. Prognostic risk factors in FL.

prognostic impact of vitamin D levels in a variety of disease processes have shown a prognostic impact that has subsequently not been shown prospectively.[71] The usefulness of vitamin D levels will likely need to be studied in a prospective setting to establish its significance.

SUMMARY

Prognostic tools in the assessment of patients with FL are constantly being refined to reflect our increasing understanding of the biological features of disease in addition to clinical features in a patient population treated using current treatment paradigms. Currently, there are a number of robust prognostic factors, but it is unclear how to best use them in conjunction to provide risk assessment at the level of each individual patient **(Fig. 1)**. Furthermore, current prognostic factors give us insight into outcomes but do not aid in decision making at an individual level (eg, wait and watch vs chemotherapy-free regimens vs chemoimmunotherapy). Future prognostic models will need to incorporate clinical information, pathology findings, genetic aberrations, and the state of the TME to fully synchronize these disparate prognostic factors. In addition, converting our prognostic information into predictive tools related to specific treatment approaches will help to decrease unnecessary physical and financial toxicity in patients.

DISCLOSURE

A.A. Patel: no disclosures. S.M. Smith: Consulting for TG Therapeutics, Bayer, Genentech, Celgene in past 12 months.

REFERENCES

1. Siegel RL, Miller KD, Jemal A. Cancer statistics, 2019. CA Cancer J Clin 2019; 69:7–34.
2. Armitage JO, Weisenburger DD. New approach to classifying Non-Hodgkin's lymphomas: clinical features of the major histologic subtypes. J Clin Oncol 1998;16:2780–95.
3. Campo E, Swerdlow SH, Harris NL, et al. The 2008 WHO classification of lymphoid neoplasms and beyond: evolving concepts and practical applications. Blood 2011;117:5019–32.
4. Tan D, Horning SJ, Hoppe RT, et al. Improvements in observed and relative survival in follicular grade 1-2 lymphoma during 4 decades: the Stanford University experience. Blood 2013;122:981–7.
5. Ott G, Katzenberger T, Lohr A, et al. Cytomorphologic, immunohistochemical, and cytogenetic profiles of follicular lymphoma: 2 types of follicular lymphoma grade 3. Blood 2002;99:3806–12.
6. Piccaluga PP, Califano A, Klein U, et al. Gene expression analysis provides a potential rationale for revising the histological grading of follicular lymphomas. Haematologica 2008;93:1033–8.
7. Horn H, Schmelter C, Leich E, et al. Follicular lymphoma grade 3B is a distinct neoplasm according to cytogenetic and immunohistochemical profiles. Haematologica 2011;96:1327–34.
8. Wahlin BE, Yri OE, Kimby E, et al. Clinical significance of the WHO grades of follicular lymphoma in a population-based cohort of 505 patients with long follow-up times: clinical significance of grading follicular lymphoma. Br J Haematol 2012;156:225–33.

9. Wahlin BE, Sundström C, Sander B, et al. Higher World Health Organization grades of follicular lymphoma correlate with better outcome in two Nordic Lymphoma Group trials of rituximab without chemotherapy. Leuk Lymphoma 2014; 55:288–95.

10. Rimsza LM, Li H, Braziel RM, et al. Impact of histological grading on survival in the SWOG S0016 follicular lymphoma cohort. Haematologica 2018;103:e151–3.

11. Summers KE, Goff LK, Wilson AG, et al. Frequency of the Bcl-2/IgH rearrangement in normal individuals: implications for the monitoring of disease in patients with follicular lymphoma. J Clin Oncol 2001;19:420–4.

12. Roulland S, Kelly RS, Morgado E, et al. t(14;18) Translocation: a predictive blood biomarker for follicular lymphoma. J Clin Oncol 2014;32:1347–55.

13. Leich E, Salaverria I, Bea S, et al. Follicular lymphomas with and without translocation t(14;18) differ in gene expression profiles and genetic alterations. Blood 2009;114:826–34.

14. Leich E, Zamo A, Horn H, et al. MicroRNA profiles of t(14;18)-negative follicular lymphoma support a late germinal center B-cell phenotype. Blood 2011;118: 5550–8.

15. Tilly H, Rossi A, Stamatoullas A, et al. Prognostic value of chromosomal abnormalities in follicular lymphoma. Blood 1994;84:1043–9.

16. Viardot A, Möller P, Högel J, et al. Clinicopathologic correlations of genomic gains and losses in follicular lymphoma. J Clin Oncol 2002;20:4523–30.

17. Mitsui T, Yokohama A, Koiso H, et al. Prognostic impact of trisomy 21 in follicular lymphoma. Br J Haematol 2019;184:570–7.

18. Qu X, Li H, Braziel RM, et al. Genomic alterations important for the prognosis in patients with follicular lymphoma treated in SWOG study S0016. Blood 2019;133: 81–93.

19. Morin RD, Mendez-Lago M, Mungall AJ, et al. Frequent mutation of histone-modifying genes in non-Hodgkin lymphoma. Nature 2011;476:298–303.

20. Okosun J, Bödör C, Wang J, et al. Integrated genomic analysis identifies recurrent mutations and evolution patterns driving the initiation and progression of follicular lymphoma. Nat Genet 2014;46:176–81.

21. Green MR. Chromatin modifying gene mutations in follicular lymphoma. Blood 2018;131:595–604.

22. Pastore A, Jurinovic V, Kridel R, et al. Integration of gene mutations in risk prognostication for patients receiving first-line immunochemotherapy for follicular lymphoma: a retrospective analysis of a prospective clinical trial and validation in a population-based registry. Lancet Oncol 2015;16:1111–22.

23. Devan J, Janikova A, Mraz M. New concepts in follicular lymphoma biology: from BCL2 to epigenetic regulators and non-coding RNAs. Semin Oncol 2018;45: 291–302.

24. Pasqualucci L, Khiabanian H, Fangazio M, et al. Genetics of follicular lymphoma transformation. Cell Rep 2014;6:130–40.

25. O'Shea D, O'Riain C, Taylor C, et al. The presence of TP53 mutation at diagnosis of follicular lymphoma identifies a high-risk group of patients with shortened time to disease progression and poorer overall survival. Blood 2008;112:3126–9.

26. Davies AJ, Lee AM, Taylor C, et al. A limited role for TP53 mutation in the transformation of follicular lymphoma to diffuse large B-cell lymphoma. Leukemia 2005;19:1459–65.

27. Alhejaily A, Day AG, Feilotter HE, et al. Inactivation of the CDKN2A tumor-suppressor gene by deletion or methylation is common at diagnosis in follicular

lymphoma and associated with poor clinical outcome. Clin Cancer Res 2014;20: 1676–86.

28. Kridel R, Chan FC, Mottok A, et al. Histological transformation and progression in follicular lymphoma: a clonal evolution study. PLoS Med 2016;13:e1002197.

29. Correia C, Schneider PA, Dai H, et al. BCL2 mutations are associated with increased risk of transformation and shortened survival in follicular lymphoma. Blood 2015;125:658–67.

30. Dave SS, Wright G, Tan B, et al. Prediction of survival in follicular lymphoma based on molecular features of tumor-infiltrating immune cells. N Engl J Med 2004;351:2159–69.

31. Scott DW, Gascoyne RD. The tumour microenvironment in B cell lymphomas. Nat Rev Cancer 2014;14:517–34.

32. Carreras J, Lopez-Guillermo A, Roncador G, et al. High numbers of tumor-infiltrating programmed cell death 1-positive regulatory lymphocytes are associated with improved overall survival in follicular lymphoma. J Clin Oncol 2009;27: 1470–6.

33. Richendollar BG, Pohlman B, Elson P, et al. Follicular programmed death 1-positive lymphocytes in the tumor microenvironment are an independent prognostic factor in follicular lymphoma. Hum Pathol 2011;42:552–7.

34. Huet S, Tesson B, Jais J-P, et al. A gene-expression profiling score for prediction of outcome in patients with follicular lymphoma: a retrospective training and validation analysis in three international cohorts. Lancet Oncol 2018;19:549–61.

35. The International Non-Hodgkin's Lymphoma Prognostic Factors Project. A predictive model for aggressive non-Hodgkin's lymphoma. N Engl J Med 1993;329:987–94.

36. López-Guillermo A, Montserrat E, Bosch F, et al. Applicability of the International Index for aggressive lymphomas to patients with low-grade lymphoma. J Clin Oncol 1994;12:1343–8.

37. Solal-Céligny P, Roy P, Colombat P, et al. Follicular lymphoma international prognostic index. Blood 2004;104:1258–65.

38. Buske C, Hoster E, Dreyling M, et al. The Follicular Lymphoma International Prognostic Index (FLIPI) separates high-risk from intermediate- or low-risk patients with advanced-stage follicular lymphoma treated front-line with rituximab and the combination of cyclophosphamide, doxorubicin, vincristine, and prednisone (R-CHOP) with respect to treatment outcome. Blood 2006;108:1504–8.

39. Nooka AK, Nabhan C, Zhou X, et al. Examination of the follicular lymphoma international prognostic index (FLIPI) in the National LymphoCare study (NLCS): a prospective US patient cohort treated predominantly in community practices. Ann Oncol 2013;24:441–8.

40. Bachy E, Maurer MJ, Habermann TM, et al. A simplified scoring system in de novo follicular lymphoma treated initially with immunochemotherapy. Blood 2018;132:49–58.

41. Federico M, Bellei M, Marcheselli L, et al. Follicular lymphoma international prognostic index 2: a new prognostic index for follicular lymphoma developed by the international follicular lymphoma prognostic factor project. J Clin Oncol 2009;27: 4555–62.

42. Lockmer S, Ren W, Brodtkorb M, et al. M7-FLIPI is not prognostic in follicular lymphoma patients with first-line rituximab chemo-free therapy. Br J Haematol 2019. https://doi.org/10.1111/bjh.16159.

43. Brice P, Bastion Y, Lepage E, et al. Comparison in low-tumor-burden follicular lymphomas between an initial no-treatment policy, prednimustine, or interferon alfa: a

randomized study from the Groupe d'Etude des Lymphomes Folliculaires. Groupe d'Etude des Lymphomes de l'Adulte. J Clin Oncol 1997;15:1110–7.

44. Zelenetz AD, Gordon LI, Abramson JS, et al. NCCN guidelines insights: B-cell lymphomas, version 3.2019. J Natl Compr Canc Netw 2019;17:651–61.

45. Meignan M, Cottereau AS, Versari A, et al. Baseline metabolic tumor volume predicts outcome in high-tumor-burden follicular lymphoma: a pooled analysis of three multicenter studies. J Clin Oncol 2016;34:3618–26.

46. St-Pierre F, Broski SM, LaPlant BR, et al. Detection of extranodal and spleen involvement by FDG-PET imaging predicts adverse survival in untreated follicular lymphoma. Am J Hematol 2019;94:786–93.

47. Schöder H, Moskowitz C. Metabolic tumor volume in lymphoma: hype or hope? J Clin Oncol 2016;34:3591–4.

48. Trotman J, Luminari S, Boussetta S, et al. Prognostic value of PET-CT after first-line therapy in patients with follicular lymphoma: a pooled analysis of central scan review in three multicentre studies. Lancet Haematol 2014;1:e17–27.

49. Cottereau AS, Versari A, Luminari S, et al. Prognostic model for high-tumor-burden follicular lymphoma integrating baseline and end-induction PET: a LYSA/FIL study. Blood 2018;131:2449–53.

50. Trotman J, Barrington SF, Belada D, et al. Prognostic value of end-of-induction PET response after first-line immunochemotherapy for follicular lymphoma (GALLIUM): secondary analysis of a randomised, phase 3 trial. Lancet Oncol 2018;19:1530–42.

51. Casulo C, Byrtek M, Dawson KL, et al. Early relapse of follicular lymphoma after rituximab plus cyclophosphamide, doxorubicin, vincristine, and prednisone defines patients at high risk for death: an analysis from the National LymphoCare Study. J Clin Oncol 2015;33:2516–22.

52. Jurinovic V, Kridel R, Staiger AM, et al. Clinicogenetic risk models predict early progression of follicular lymphoma after first-line immunochemotherapy. Blood 2016;128:1112–20.

53. Moccia A, Schar S, Hayoz S, et al. Predictive value of POD24 validation in follicular lymphoma patients initially treated with chemotherapy-free regimens in a pooled analysis of three randomized trials of the Swiss group for clinical cancer research (SAKK). Hematol Oncol 2019;37:111–2.

54. Maurer MJ, Bachy E, Ghesquières H, et al. Early event status informs subsequent outcome in newly diagnosed follicular lymphoma. Am J Hematol 2016;91:1096–101.

55. Cheson BD, Chua N, Mayer J, et al. Overall survival benefit in patients with rituximab-refractory indolent non-Hodgkin lymphoma who received obinutuzumab plus bendamustine induction and obinutuzumab maintenance in the GADOLIN study. J Clin Oncol 2018;36:2259–66.

56. Gopal AK, Kahl BS, de Vos S, et al. PI3Kδ inhibition by idelalisib in patients with relapsed indolent lymphoma. N Engl J Med 2014;370:1008–18.

57. Shi Q, Flowers CR, Hiddemann W, et al. Thirty-month complete response as a surrogate end point in first-line follicular lymphoma therapy: an individual patient-level analysis of multiple randomized trials. J Clin Oncol 2017;35:552–60.

58. Delfau-Larue M-H, van der Gucht A, Dupuis J, et al. Total metabolic tumor volume, circulating tumor cells, cell-free DNA: distinct prognostic value in follicular lymphoma. Blood Adv 2018;2:807–16.

59. Rossi D, Spina V, Bruscaggin A, et al. Liquid biopsy in lymphoma. Haematologica 2019;104:648–52.

60. Zohren F, Bruns I, Pechtel S, et al. Prognostic value of circulating Bcl-2/IgH levels in patients with follicular lymphoma receiving first-line immunochemotherapy. Blood 2015;126:1407–14.
61. Pott C, Hoster E, Kehden B, et al. Minimal residual disease response at end of induction and during maintenance correlates with updated outcome in the Phase III GALLIUM study of obinutuzumab- or rituximab-based immunochemotherapy in previously untreated follicular lymphoma patients. Blood 2018;132:396.
62. Pulsoni A, Della Starza I, Cappelli LV, et al. Minimal residual disease monitoring in early stage follicular lymphoma can predict prognosis and drive treatment with rituximab after radiotherapy. Br J Haematol 2019. https://doi.org/10.1111/bjh.16125.
63. Bastion Y, Sebban C, Berger F, et al. Incidence, predictive factors, and outcome of lymphoma transformation in follicular lymphoma patients. J Clin Oncol 1997; 15:1587–94.
64. Al-Tourah AJ, Gill KK, Chhanabhai M, et al. Population-based analysis of incidence and outcome of transformed non-Hodgkin's lymphoma. J Clin Oncol 2008;26:5165–9.
65. Wagner-Johnston ND, Link BK, Byrtek M, et al. Outcomes of transformed follicular lymphoma in the modern era: a report from the National LymphoCare Study (NLCS). Blood 2015;126:851–7.
66. Sarkozy C, Trneny M, Xerri L, et al. Risk factors and outcomes for patients with follicular lymphoma who had histologic transformation after response to first-line immunochemotherapy in the PRIMA trial. J Clin Oncol 2016;34:2575–82.
67. Freeman CL, Kridel R, Moccia AA, et al. Early progression after bendamustine-rituximab is associated with high risk of transformation in advanced stage follicular lymphoma. Blood 2019;134:761–4.
68. Federico M, Caballero Barrigón MD, Marcheselli L, et al. Rituximab and the risk of transformation of follicular lymphoma: a retrospective pooled analysis. Lancet Haematol 2018;5:e359–67.
69. Kelly JL, Salles G, Goldman B, et al. Low serum Vitamin D levels are associated with inferior survival in follicular lymphoma: a prospective evaluation in SWOG and LYSA studies. J Clin Oncol 2015;33:1482–90.
70. Tracy SI, Maurer MJ, Witzig TE, et al. Vitamin D insufficiency is associated with an increased risk of early clinical failure in follicular lymphoma. Blood Cancer J 2017; 7:e595.
71. Lucas A, Wolf M. Vitamin D and health outcomes: then came the randomized clinical trials. JAMA 2019. https://doi.org/10.1001/jama.2019.17302.

Initial Treatment of Early Stage and Low Tumor Burden Follicular Lymphoma

Jonathon B. Cohen, MD, MS[a], Brad S. Kahl, MD[b],*

KEYWORDS

- Follicular lymphoma • Low tumor burden • Rituximab • Watchful waiting
- Early stage • Non-Hodgkin lymphoma

KEY POINTS

- Many patients diagnosed with follicular lymphoma have early stage disease or asymptomatic advanced-stage disease with low tumor burden.
- Patients with limited-stage disease can potentially be cured with radiation therapy and should be considered for this approach.
- Patients with low tumor burden and advanced-stage disease can likely be observed but a single-agent rituximab can delay the time to cytotoxic chemotherapy may result in improved quality of life.

INTRODUCTION

Up to 30% of patients with follicular lymphoma (FL) have stage I or II disease at diagnosis and their management approach and expected prognosis often differs from patients with advanced-stage disease.[1] In addition, many patients who do have advanced-stage disease have a low tumor burden that permits observation or de-escalation of the intensity of front-line therapy. As a result, staging to assess extent of disease and overall tumor burden is a critical aspect of the evaluation of a new patient. In this article, we describe methods used to assess tumor burden and review the data describing optimal approaches to patients with low tumor burden and/or limited-stage disease.

DEFINITION OF LOW TUMOR BURDEN FOLLICULAR LYMPHOMA

Although it can sometimes be readily apparent by clinical assessment whether a patient has a significant burden of disease or not, standardized criteria are needed to

[a] Department of Hematology and Medical Oncology, Emory University – Winship Cancer Institute, 1365 Clifton Road, Suite B400, Atlanta, GA 30322, USA; [b] Department of Medicine, Washington University School of Medicine, 660 South Euclid Avenue, Campus Box 8056, St Louis, MO 63110, USA
* Corresponding author.
E-mail address: bkahl@wustl.edu

Hematol Oncol Clin N Am 34 (2020) 663–672
https://doi.org/10.1016/j.hoc.2020.02.003
0889-8588/20/© 2020 Elsevier Inc. All rights reserved.

inform guidelines and clinical trial development. The most commonly used guidelines were developed in a French study led by the Groupe d'Etude des Lymphomes Folliculaires (GELF) comparing watchful waiting, prednimustine, and interferon-α in patients who met the criteria for having a low tumor burden (**Box 1**).[2] There was no significant difference in overall survival (OS) regardless of treatment approach, and patients who were observed off therapy remained off treatment for a median of 24 months. Although these criteria were published greater than 20 years ago, they have been used frequently in the management of patients on clinical trials and in common clinical practice and are included in current guidelines to determine therapy. In subsequent years, modifications to these criteria have been assessed, although many current studies continue to rely on the original GELF criteria to inform treatment selection.

In addition to baseline tumor burden defined by GELF, other studies have relied on identification of high-risk FL by use of additional clinical/laboratory criteria. The Follicular Lymphoma International Prognostic Index (FLIPI) includes age, lactate dehydrogenase, hemoglobin, presence of advanced-stage disease (stage III and IV), and number of involved nodal areas to develop a score that has been used to identify low (0,1), intermediate (2), and high (3–5) risk patient groups with 10-year OS ranging from 71% for low-risk patients to 36% for high-risk patients.[3] Although this index was not specifically designed to inform the need for treatment, subsequent studies have identified a clear association of patients with intermediate- and high-risk FLIPI scores with tumor burden according to GELF criteria.[4,5] There have been attempts to improve the prognostic value of the FLIPI including the FLIPI2, which used β^2-microglobulin, bone marrow involvement, longest diameter of the largest involved node greater than 6 cm, hemoglobin, and age to construct an updated model.[6] More recently, the m7-FLIPI has integrated mutational analysis for seven genes with the FLIPI to attempt to generate a more comprehensive approach to risk stratification.[7] Although these prognostic models frequently are associated with tumor burden, it remains unclear whether a patient with a high-risk FLIPI should automatically be treated as if they have a high tumor burden, and often those cases are best managed by a thorough evaluation of the patient, their symptoms, and comorbidities when determining a treatment approach.

Box 1
The original Groupe d'Etude des Lymphomes Folliculaires criteria for determination of tumor burden in untreated follicular lymphoma

Nodal or extranodal tumor mass >7 cm

Involvement of at least 3 nodal sites, each with a diameter >3 cm

Presence of any B symptoms

Splenomegaly

Compression syndrome related to disease

Pleural effusion or ascites

Leukemic phase (>5.0 × 10^9/L circulating lymphoma cells)

Cytopenias (neutrophils <1.0 × 10^9/L and/or platelets <100 × 10^9/L)

Data from Brice P, Bastion Y, Lepage E, et al: Comparison in low-tumor-burden follicular lymphomas between an initial no-treatment policy, prednimustine, or interferon alfa: a randomized study from the Groupe d'Etude des Lymphomes Folliculaires. Groupe d'Etude des Lymphomes de l'Adulte. J Clin Oncol 15:1110-7, 1997.

STUDIES IN FOLLICULAR LYMPHOMA WITH LIMITED-STAGE DISEASE

FL is typically considered incurable but patients presenting with a more limited disease stage may experience prolonged (occasionally indefinite) disease remissions. In these cases, initiating therapy at the time of diagnosis is often indicated to provide the opportunity for an indefinite treatment-free interval, often after a short course of radiation therapy (RT) alone. Some of the initial studies evaluating the management of early stage FL identified RT as potentially curative in that setting, and selected studies evaluating the role of RT alone in early stage FL are highlighted in **Table 1**.[8] It is important to recognize that the ability to stage patients accurately has improved dramatically with the availability of PET in conjunction with computed tomography (CT). PET/CT has likely resulted in the upstaging of patients who would have previously been considered to have stage I or II and it is not surprising that more recent studies have shown even better long-term progression-free survival (PFS) and OS for patients who truly have limited-stage disease.

One large study (TROG 99.03) of patients with stage I-II FL included 150 patients enrolled from 2000 to 2012 who received either 30-Gy involved field RT or involved field RT plus cyclophosphamide, vincristine, and prednisone with rituximab added after 2006.[9] This study spanned the years when PET/CT would have been adopted and was not a requirement for all patients. After nearly 10 years of follow-up, the 10-year PFS for radiation alone was 41% compared with 59% for chemotherapy plus RT. There was no significant difference in OS between these two approaches (87% and 95% at 10 years). The appropriate RT dose to use in this setting is likely between 24 and 30 Gy based on the published TROG study and a randomized trial from the United Kingdom, which compared the use of 40 to 45 Gy with 24 Gy in patients with indolent non-Hodgkin lymphoma (NHL).[10] Response rates were equivalent and there was no significant difference in within-filed progression. As a result, 24 Gy is likely appropriate in this setting and may decrease toxicities associated with a higher dose.

Additional retrospective assessments have also evaluated the role of RT and other treatment modalities in the management of early stage FL. One of the first studies presented from Stanford included long-term follow-up for patients with early stage FL treated with RT with follow-up up to 31 years (median, 7.7 years). In this series, which included patients with only stage I or II disease (using available staging techniques at

Table 1
Outcomes for patients with early stage FL who received RT alone

Study	N	PET/CT Staging?	PFS	OS
MacManus et al,[9] 2018	75	Some patients	10 y: 41%	10 y: 86%
Manus & Hoppe,[8] 1996	177	No	10 y: 40%	10 y: 64%
			20 y: 37%	20 y: 35%
Tobin et al,[11] 2019	171	Yes	5 y: 68%	5 y: 93%
Ng et al,[12] 2019	47	Yes	5 y: 78%	5 y: 97%
Brady et al,[13] 2019	512	Yes	5 y FFP: 69%	5 y: 96%
Friedberg et al,[14] 2012	206	Yes	Median: 72 mo	—
Guckenberger et al,[23] 2012	86	No	10 y FFP: 58%	10 y: 64%
			15 y FFP: 56%	15 y: 50%

Abbreviations: CT, computed tomography; FFP, freedom from progression; PFS, progression-free survival.
Data from Refs.[8,9,11–14,23]

the time of diagnosis), 37% of patients remained relapse-free at 20 years, and only 5/47 patients who remained relapse-free at 10 years subsequently relapse.[8]

Tobin and colleagues[11] recently published a multicenter study from Australia and Canada including 365 patients, most of whom (n = 171) received RT alone. There was no significant difference between patients receiving RT alone or chemotherapy with regards to PFS or OS with a median follow-up of 45 months. During this observation period, 25% of patients treated with RT alone experienced disease progression. An additional series of 47 patients with early stage FL treated with RT between 2000 and 2011 from Australia found excellent long-term PFS.[12] When staged with a PET/CT, the 5-year PFS for patients with stage I was 84% and for stage II was 60%. Seven-year OS was 91% for all patients.

The International Lymphoma Radiation Oncology Group (ILROG) published a large series of 512 patients with early stage FL as determined by PET/CT who received RT alone.[13] The 5-year freedom from progression was 69%, and 5-year OS was 96%. Extent of radiation field did not seem to impact outcome, although patients with stage II FL had an inferior freedom from progression compared with patients with stage I.

Although several studies have identified a sizable group of patients who can enjoy prolonged remissions with early stage FL treated with RT, additional studies have investigated the role of incorporating systemic treatment, including the case of grade 3 FL. For example, in 55 patients with limited-stage grade 3 FL treated at MD Anderson Cancer Center, outcomes were superior for patients who received systemic treatment followed by RT when compared with RT alone (P = .003), although there was no difference in OS. These findings would suggest that patients with grade 3 FL may benefit from an approach comparable with an aggressive NHL where chemotherapy is frequently administered before RT to involved areas.

Friedberg and colleagues[14] reported outcomes for patients with stage I FL in the National LymphoCare study, including those patients who were "rigorously staged" with a bone marrow biopsy and either CT or PET/CT. Of these 206 patients, there were a variety of treatment approaches including observation (17%), rituximab monotherapy (12%), rituximab plus chemotherapy (28%), radiation (27%), and RT plus systemic treatment (13%). Patients who received chemotherapy or systemic therapy plus radiation had significantly improved PFS compared with those receiving radiation alone. There was no difference between all groups with regards to OS.

MANAGEMENT APPROACHES TO ADVANCED-STAGE FOLLICULAR LYMPHOMA WITH LIMITED TUMOR BURDEN
Outcomes from Watchful Waiting Versus Immediate Treatment

Unlike patients with limited-stage FL, the incidence of cure in patients with advanced-stage FL is low. However, most patients with advanced-stage FL experience a prolonged OS, often approaching that of unaffected age-matched patients. As a result, it is critical to consider the patient's overall life expectancy, possible short- and long-term toxicities of treatment, and how the underlying disease and the possible treatment may impact a patient's lifestyle or quality of life when deciding to start therapy in patients with low tumor burden.

Several studies have investigated the impact of treatment initiation versus watchful waiting in patients with low tumor burden FL. The original study that established the GELF criteria for determining low tumor burden was published in 1997 and reported results of a randomized trial comparing watchful waiting, prednimustine, or interferon-α.[2] Although the time to receiving additional treatment was shorter in patients who initiated a watchful waiting program compared with those started on treatment, there was no significant difference in 5-OS (78% for watchful waiting, 70% for prednimustine, and 84% for interferon-α). Although these therapy approaches are not typically used in the modern era, this study has served as the basis for selection of watchful waiting as an appropriate treatment approach for patients meeting the criteria spelled out in the study.

Despite these findings, it has remained unclear whether incorporation of modern therapies may impact the selected approach for patients with low tumor burden FL diagnosed currently. Specifically, rituximab has changed the management of all B-cell lymphomas in the past 20 years and has been evaluated on several occasions in patients with low tumor burden FL.

Ardeshna and colleagues[15] published a randomized study in which patients were assigned to watchful waiting, an abbreviated course of rituximab 375 mg/m^2 for 4 weekly doses, or 4 weekly doses followed by 12 maintenance doses administered every 2 months for 2 years. Ultimately the study was amended to be a two-arm study and the induction-alone arm was discontinued once the role of maintenance rituximab in FL was established. The primary end point of the study was the time to new treatment, which could be any therapy (systemic or RT) received after randomization (not including the study-prescribed rituximab for those randomized to those arms). The median time to start of new treatment was 31 months in the watchful waiting group, whereas it was not reached in the rituximab induction plus maintenance group, and at 3 years, 46% of patients in watchful waiting had not needed new treatment compared with 88% in the rituximab group. There was no significant OS benefit by treating with rituximab. Subsequent studies (ie, E4402) would further explore the importance of maintenance rituximab in low tumor burden FL. Although this study suggests that initiation of chemotherapy is delayed by using single-agent rituximab in asymptomatic patients with low tumor burden FL, the lack of an OS benefit implies that patients may generally safely defer initiation of treatment.

In addition to these prospective studies, several retrospective series have evaluated the safety of watchful waiting in patients with low tumor burden FL. Identification of a patient managed with watchful waiting can sometimes be challenging in the setting of a retrospective study because it is not always clear what the intention of the treating physician may have been. One such analysis, the F2-study, initially developed to validate the FLIPI score, included nearly 1100 newly diagnosed patients with FL, 134 of whom were initially monitored without treatment (including 107 ultimately eligible for analysis).[4] For this study, watchful waiting was defined as initiation of therapy at least 3 months after initial diagnosis. Within this group, the median time of observation before initiation of therapy was 55 months, and among those who initiated treatment, the median time to treatment initiation was 14 months. In a multivariate analysis evaluating time to initiation of treatment, only presence of greater than four nodal sites was associated with a shorter time to initiation of treatment. The 5-year OS was 87% and did not differ significantly from those patients in the study who initiated therapy at the time of diagnosis (87%).

A Danish population-based study included patients with stage III-IVA disease who were observed for at least 90 days after initial diagnosis and identified 286 eligible patients diagnosed between 2000 and 2011, which comprised 34% of all patients diagnosed with advanced-stage FL during this time period in Denmark.[16] The 5-year OS for patients on watchful waiting was 83%, compared with 78% for patients who received initial therapy, although this study included patients regardless of baseline tumor burden. The authors conducted an additional analysis evaluating the average loss of residual lifetime for watchful waiting patients (compared with matched, unaffected control subjects from the population) and found that the average loss of residual lifetime was 6 years. The 10-year risk of dying from lymphoma in this group of patients was 13%.

A Japanese study included the same 3-month cutoff to identify patients treated with watchful waiting and evaluated 348 patients, 101 of whom were managed with watchful waiting.[17] Among the patients who ultimately received treatment during the period of observation (45% of watchful waiting patients), the median time to treatment was 16 months. The most common indications for treatment were either objective evidence of progressive disease or the development of symptoms related to the lymphoma. There was no significant difference in OS between those patients receiving immediate treatment versus watchful waiting, and there was no difference in rate of transformation. There were 20 patients who met criteria for high tumor burden in the watchful waiting group, and these patients had a similar OS and rate of transformation when compared with the high tumor burden patients in the immediate treatment group, suggesting that although these objective criteria may be helpful for appropriately and objectively describing patient groups, there likely remains some space for personalized clinical assessment when determining the most appropriate management strategy for an individual patient.

The National LymphoCare Study evaluated the role of watchful waiting as compared with active treatment of patients throughout the United States who had newly diagnosed stage II-IV FL.[18] Of 1754 patients included in the series, 22% were managed with watchful waiting, 17% received rituximab monotherapy, and 61% received rituximab plus chemotherapy. The early use of treatment had no impact on OS (regardless of rituximab monotherapy or rituximab-chemotherapy use). However, patients who received chemotherapy had a lower rate of subsequent transformation, and patients receiving therapy for any type had a longer time to a new treatment when compared with patients managed with watchful waiting. Median time to initiation of a new treatment was 2.3 years for patients engaged in watchful waiting, 4.4 years for patients receiving rituximab monotherapy, and not reached for patients receiving chemotherapy. Rituximab monotherapy also resulted in a longer time to initiation of chemotherapy when compared with watchful waiting.

Rituximab Monotherapy Treatment Strategies

Although there does not seem to be a survival benefit to early initiation of treatment in patients with low tumor burden FL, there are other potential indications to start treatment, including desires to delay more intensive therapy, patient/physician preference, and the potential to use effective therapies with limited toxicity to potentially improve the course of the disease.

E4402 (RESORT) evaluated two treatment approaches using rituximab monotherapy for patients with low tumor burden FL (**Fig. 1**).[19] In this trial, patients with grade 1 or 2 FL who were classified as having low tumor burden by GELF were randomized to one of two rituximab treatment schedules: retreatment versus maintenance. In both arms, patients received 4 weekly doses of rituximab monotherapy. Those assigned to retreatment discontinued therapy at that time and were retreated with rituximab for 4 weeks at the time of each successive progression until treatment failure, defined as no response to rituximab, progression within 26 weeks, initiation of alternative therapy, or inability to complete the planned treatment. Patients assigned to maintenance rituximab received one dose of rituximab every 13 weeks until treatment failure. Of note, any progressive disease that occurred between maintenance doses was considered a treatment failure.

There were no significant differences between treatment approaches with regards to time to treatment failure. Among the patients assigned to rituximab retreatment,

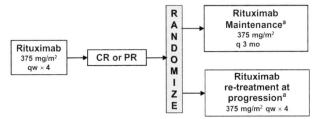

Fig. 1. Trial schema for RESORT trial evaluating two rituximab treatment schedules in untreated low tumor burden indolent non-Hodgkin lymphoma. [a] Continue until treatment failure, defined as: (1) no response to retreatment or PD within 6 months of rituximab, (2) initiation of cytotoxic therapy, or (3) inability to complete prescribed treatment. CR, complete response; PD, progressive disease; PR, partial response; qw, every week.

the median response duration to the first four-dose induction treatment was 34.4 months, and those who required a second course of rituximab had a median response duration of 18.5 months. There was no difference in OS between the two group (94% at 5 years for both arms). The rate of remaining free of cytotoxic therapy at 3 years was higher in the maintenance arm (95%) compared with the retreatment arm (84%). However, this benefit came at a cost of requiring more rituximab in the maintenance arm when compared with the retreatment arm.

Cost Effectiveness and Quality of Life in Low Tumor Burden Follicular Lymphoma

Although OS and time to subsequent treatment are clinically meaningful end points, especially for an individual patient, it is important to consider additional outcomes related to the choice of initial approach for patients with untreated FL with a low tumor burden who are asymptomatic. In the United Kingdom, one study evaluated the overall cost of treatment based on one of three initial approaches: watchful waiting, rituximab induction alone, or rituximab induction followed by maintenance.[20] This analysis accounted for subsequent treatments including chemotherapy-based treatments and the use of autologous stem cell transplantation for patients with relapsed disease who are less than 65 years of age. The use of rituximab induction (without maintenance) was the most cost-effective approach within the United Kingdom health care system, and watchful waiting was the least cost-effective, suggesting that the delayed need for combination chemotherapy and/or more costly intensive approaches outweighs the potential benefit seen in delaying initial rituximab treatment. A similar analysis in Canada found the same result: rituximab induction (without maintenance) is more cost-effective over a patient's lifetime than rituximab induction plus maintenance or a watchful waiting approach.[21]

The RESORT trial incorporated assessments of illness-related anxiety and general anxiety, health-related quality of life, and other patient-reported outcomes as secondary objectives assessing the differences between two rituximab treatment approaches for low tumor burden FL.[22] Patients participating in this study completed measures at the time of randomization after the 4 weeks of rituximab induction, and then at predetermined timepoints up to 4 years after the baseline assessment. These were also completed at the time of rituximab failure. There were no significant differences in any of the patient-reported outcome measures including quality of life, illness-related anxiety, or general anxiety, indicating that in this setting, the use of maintenance rituximab does not provide any benefit to patients with regards to anxiety about their illness.

In the Ardeshna trial that compared watchful waiting with initiation of rituximab for patients with low tumor burden, quality of life was also included as a secondary end point.[15] There were several identified differences between arms, all of which favored the rituximab when compared with watchful waiting, including an improvement in mental adjustment to cancer between baseline and Month 7, worsened illness coping style in the watchful waiting group, and a decrease level of worry about the need for treatment or more treatment in the treatment group compared with watchful waiting.

SUMMARY AND RECOMMENDATIONS

Fortunately, most patients with early stage and/or low tumor burden FL enjoy a prolonged life expectancy and benefit from many currently available treatments, which are becoming increasingly tolerable. As a result, it is difficult to identify therapies that result in prolonged OS for this low-risk group of patients. Patients should therefore be offered treatments that are in line with their personalized goals (ie, delaying intensive therapy, possibility of long-term remission/cure).

In early stage FL, RT alone results in remission duration of greater than 5 years for most patients, and even with follow-up of 10 to 20 years, roughly 40% of patients remain remission-free, suggesting that when feasible, this should be considered for most patients with early stage FL as a possible curative option. Although the precise radiation dose for use in this setting has not been defined, doses of 24 Gy have been compared with higher doses (40–45 Gy) in indolent NHL with no apparent decrease in efficacy. We suggest consideration of an abbreviated course of chemotherapy followed by RT for patients with grade 3 FL given the MD Anderson Cancer Center experience and the concern for clinical behavior comparable with diffuse large B-cell lymphoma, where combination of chemotherapy with RT is often appropriate in patients with limited-stage disease.

In patients with advanced-stage disease with low tumor burden, the decision to initiate treatment is often more complicated. Many patients are reluctant to undergo treatment if it will not result in improved survival, whereas other patients are uncomfortable with the idea of watchful waiting. In these cases, the knowledge of a developing disease process and anxiety regarding its progression often outweighs any cost or toxicity benefit achieved by holding off on treatment. In fact, several studies have confirmed that watchful waiting may be less cost effective and associated with worsened adjustment of patients to their illness over time. As a result, it is critical to discuss treatment versus watchful waiting with each patient, taking into account their specific disease presentation and feeling regarding treatment.

When treatment is indicated, rituximab monotherapy is likely the most appropriate choice in many cases, and maintenance rituximab is unlikely to result in improved quality of life, cost-effectiveness, time to treatment failure, or OS. The one potential benefit for maintenance rituximab in low tumor burden FL may be to prolong the time before the need for cytotoxic therapy, but in the current era where novel, noncytotoxic agents continue to emerge, this end point may become less meaningful. We would recommend incorporating maintenance in low tumor burden FL for those patients who would be ineligible for more aggressive treatments based on underlying comorbidities. We do not recommend use of additional therapies (ie, oral targeted agents) in this setting outside of a clinical trial because the role of indefinite treatment in patients with low tumor burden FL is not well-established and the expected prolonged OS without such treatments makes it difficult to justify the frequently encountered chronic low-grade toxicities associated with such therapies.

In summary, patients with early stage and low tumor burden FL require a personalized approach to treatment with the goal of minimizing treatment-related toxicities in this low-risk patient population while maximizing the time off intensive therapies. Patients in this subgroup should continue to be evaluated in ongoing investigations to potentially identify well-tolerated approaches that could result in possible cure and/or marked prolongation of remission beyond current expectations. Given the prolonged OS enjoyed by patients who completed watchful waiting and/or limited intensity treatment, any future trials in this space should include quality of life and toxicity-related end points because these important determinants of success of future treatments.

DISCLOSURE

Dr B.S. Kahl reports consulting activities for Genentech.

REFERENCES

1. Friedberg JW, Taylor MD, Cerhan JR, et al. Follicular lymphoma in the United States: first report of the National LymphoCare Study. J Clin Oncol 2009;27: 1202–8.
2. Brice P, Bastion Y, Lepage E, et al. Comparison in low-tumor-burden follicular lymphomas between an initial no-treatment policy, prednimustine, or interferon alfa: a randomized study from the Groupe d'Etude des Lymphomes Folliculaires. Groupe d'Etude des Lymphomes de l'Adulte. J Clin Oncol 1997;15:1110–7.
3. Solal-Celigny P, Roy P, Colombat P, et al. Follicular lymphoma international prognostic index. Blood 2004;104:1258–65.
4. Solal-Céligny P, Bellei M, Marcheselli L, et al. Watchful waiting in low–tumor burden follicular lymphoma in the rituximab era: results of an F2-study database. J Clin Oncol 2012;30:3848–53.
5. Nooka AK, Nabhan C, Zhou X, et al. Examination of the follicular lymphoma international prognostic index (FLIPI) in the National LymphoCare study (NLCS): a prospective US patient cohort treated predominantly in community practices. Ann Oncol 2013;24:441–8.
6. Federico M, Bellei M, Marcheselli L, et al. Follicular lymphoma international prognostic index 2: a new prognostic index for follicular lymphoma developed by the international follicular lymphoma prognostic factor project. J Clin Oncol 2009;27: 4555–62.
7. Pastore A, Jurinovic V, Kridel R, et al. Integration of gene mutations in risk prognostication for patients receiving first-line immunochemotherapy for follicular lymphoma: a retrospective analysis of a prospective clinical trial and validation in a population-based registry. Lancet Oncol 2015;16:1111–22.
8. Manus MPM, Hoppe RT. Is radiotherapy curative for stage I and II low-grade follicular lymphoma? Results of a long-term follow-up study of patients treated at Stanford University. J Clin Oncol 1996;14:1282–90.
9. MacManus M, Fisher R, Roos D, et al. Randomized trial of systemic therapy after involved-field radiotherapy in patients with early-stage follicular lymphoma: TROG 99.03. J Clin Oncol 2018;36:2918–25.
10. Lowry L, Smith P, Qian W, et al. Reduced dose radiotherapy for local control in non-Hodgkin lymphoma: a randomised phase III trial. Radiother Oncol 2011; 100:86–92.

11. Tobin JWD, Rule G, Colvin K, et al. Outcomes of stage I/II follicular lymphoma in the PET era: an international study from the Australian Lymphoma Alliance. Blood Adv 2019;3:2804–11.
12. Ng SP, Khor R, Bressel M, et al. Outcome of patients with early-stage follicular lymphoma staged with 18F-fluorodeoxyglucose (FDG) positron emission tomography (PET) and treated with radiotherapy alone. Eur J Nucl Med Mol Imaging 2019;46:80–6.
13. Brady JL, Binkley MS, Hajj C, et al. Definitive radiotherapy for localized follicular lymphoma staged by 18F-FDG PET-CT: a collaborative study by ILROG. Blood 2019;133:237–45.
14. Friedberg JW, Byrtek M, Link BK, et al. Effectiveness of first-line management strategies for stage I follicular lymphoma: analysis of the National LymphoCare Study. J Clin Oncol 2012;30:3368–75.
15. Ardeshna KM, Qian W, Smith P, et al. Rituximab versus a watch-and-wait approach in patients with advanced-stage, asymptomatic, non-bulky follicular lymphoma: an open-label randomised phase 3 trial. Lancet Oncol 2014;15: 424–35.
16. El-Galaly TC, Bilgrau AE, de Nully Brown P, et al. A population-based study of prognosis in advanced stage follicular lymphoma managed by watch and wait. Br J Haematol 2015;169:435–44.
17. Yuda S, Maruyama D, Maeshima AM, et al. Influence of the watch and wait strategy on clinical outcomes of patients with follicular lymphoma in the rituximab era. Ann Hematol 2016;95:2017–22.
18. Nastoupil LJ, Sinha R, Byrtek M, et al. Outcomes following watchful waiting for stage II-IV follicular lymphoma patients in the modern era. Br J Haematol 2016; 172:724–34.
19. Kahl BS, Hong F, Williams ME, et al. Rituximab extended schedule or re-treatment trial for low-tumor burden follicular lymphoma: eastern cooperative oncology group protocol e4402. J Clin Oncol 2014;32:3096–102.
20. Prettyjohns M, Hoskin P, McNamara C, et al. The cost-effectiveness of immediate treatment or watch and wait with deferred chemotherapy for advanced asymptomatic follicular lymphoma. Br J Haematol 2018;180:52–9.
21. Prica A, Chan K, Cheung M. Frontline rituximab monotherapy induction versus a watch and wait approach for asymptomatic advanced-stage follicular lymphoma: a cost-effectiveness analysis. Cancer 2015;121:2637–45.
22. Wagner LI, Zhao F, Hong F, et al. Anxiety and health-related quality of life among patients with low-tumor burden non-Hodgkin lymphoma randomly assigned to two different rituximab dosing regimens: results from ECOG trial E4402 (RESORT). J Clin Oncol 2015;33:740–8.
23. Guckenberger M, Alexandrow N, Flentje M. Radiotherapy alone for stage I-III low grade follicular lymphoma: long-term outcome and comparison of extended field and total nodal irradiation. Radiat Oncol 2012;7:103.

Initial Treatment of High Tumor Burden Follicular Lymphoma

Ciara L. Freeman, MB BCh, MSc, FRCPathUK, FRCPC*,
Laurie H. Sehn, MD, MPH

KEYWORDS

- Follicular lymphoma • Advanced stage • Immunochemotherapy
- High tumor burden

KEY POINTS

- All newly diagnosed patients with follicular lymphoma should be carefully investigated to stage their disease and ascertain whether they have high or low tumor burden.
- Patients meeting the criteria for high tumor burden should be considered for immediate initiation of systemic therapy if clinically appropriate.
- Immunochemotherapy remains the standard upfront therapy for high tumor burden follicular lymphoma, which includes an anti-CD20 monoclonal antibody and chemotherapy (most commonly bendamustine, CHOP [cyclophosphamide, doxorubicin, vincristine and prednisone], or CVP [cyclophosphamide, vincristine and prednisone]).
- Patients can expect excellent outcomes in the modern treatment era with overall survival estimates of 80% at 10 years; however, those who experience transformation or early-treatment failure represent a high-risk population.

WHAT CONSTITUTES HIGH TUMOR BURDEN IN PATIENTS WITH FOLLICULAR LYMPHOMA

Most newly diagnosed patients with follicular lymphoma (FL) will have evidence of advanced-stage disease at presentation. Within the observational National Lympho-Care Study including more than 2000 patients with FL, 69% of patients were identified as having advanced-stage disease at diagnosis, and 68% of this cohort were immediately treated with some form of rituximab-containing systemic therapy.[1]

Because initial management is largely dictated by disease burden and the presence of lymphoma-related symptoms, a detailed history and careful staging evaluation are critical. Patients meeting the criteria for high tumor burden generally require immediate

BC Cancer Centre for Lymphoid Cancer, The University of British Columbia, 600 West 10th Avenue, Vancouver, British Columbia V5Z 4E6, Canada
* Corresponding author.
E-mail address: Ciara.freeman@bccancer.bc.ca

Hematol Oncol Clin N Am 34 (2020) 673–687
https://doi.org/10.1016/j.hoc.2020.02.004
0889-8588/20/Crown Copyright © 2020 Published by Elsevier Inc. All rights reserved.

and definitive therapy and are not appropriate candidates for expectant management ("watch and wait").[2]

There are no universally established criteria for high tumor burden disease, but criteria designated within clinical trials may serve as a general guide for clinical practice (**Table 1**). The Groupe D'Etudes des Lymphomes Folliculaires (GELF) criteria, established in the late 1990s, were used to allocate patients within clinical trials, separating those with low versus high tumor burden disease into different treatment approaches.[3,4] These criteria have been modified over time, but include measurement of clinical symptoms, tumor mass size, organ compromise, and cell counts reflecting higher disease burden. More recently, additional laboratory parameters, such as elevated lactate dehydrogenase (LDH) and beta-2-microglobulin (B2M) levels, have been used as surrogate markers of disease burden and also feature within clinical prognostication scoring systems for newly diagnosed patients with FL.[5–7] Although the Follicular Lymphoma International Prognostic Index (FLIPI) score and FLIPI-2 score are prognostic for patients with FL, they were not designed to establish high tumor burden disease or need for treatment.[5,8,9]

THE OPTIMAL STAGING: TO PET OR NOT TO PET?

Careful assessment at initial diagnosis is critical to establish stage and level of tumor burden, as well as for prognostication and treatment planning.[2,13] History should

Table 1
Comparison of criteria used for the purposes of clinical trials to consider patients "high tumor burden"

Original GELF Criteria 1997[4]	British National Lymphoma Investigation Criteria 2003[10]	Salles et al,[11] 2011; Marcus et al,[12] 2017
Patients must meet ≥1 criterion	• B symptoms or severe pruritus	• Largest nodal or EN site ≥7 cm
• Any nodal or extranodal (EN) tumor mass >7 cm in diameter	• Life-threatening organ involvement	• Involvement of ≥3 nodal sites >3 cm
• Involvement of ≥3 nodal sites ≥3 cm	• Rapid disease progression during preceding 3 mo	• Presence of systemic symptoms
• Presence of any systemic or B symptoms	• Marrow infiltration causing cytopenias	• Organ compression
• Pleural or peritoneal serous effusion (irrespective of cell content)	• Localized bone lesions	• Ascites or pleural effusion
• Splenic enlargement with inferior margin below the umbilical line	• Renal infiltration	• Symptomatic spleen enlargement
• Compression syndrome (ureteral, orbital, gastrointestinal)	• Macroscopic liver involvement	• Eastern Cooperative Oncology Group (ECOG) performance status of >1
• Leukemic phase (>5.0 × 10⁹/L circulating malignant cells)		• LDH or B2M > Upper Limit of Normal
• Cytopenia (granulocyte count <1.0 × 10⁹/L and/or platelets <100 × 10⁹/L)		

Data from Refs.[4,10–12]

probe for the presence of B symptoms, constitutional upset, or significant pruritus. Physical examination should evaluate for the presence of peripheral lymphadenopathy, hepatosplenomegaly, or serous effusions. Laboratory workup should include baseline hematological parameters, markers of tumor burden (LDH, B2M), and serology. If there is suggestion of an elevated lymphocyte count, peripheral blood immunophenotyping may identify the presence of a circulating clone. Bone marrow evaluation should be routinely considered in all patients for staging accuracy and prognostic relevance.[6,7] Computed tomography (CT) scanning from neck to pelvis has been commonly used to assess sites of involvement and tumor mass dimensions. However, recent data demonstrate the utility of fluorodeoxyglucose (FDG) -PET for both staging and response assessment.

Since the publication of the revised Lugano criteria, pretreatment evaluation with FDG-PET has been recommended for FL given its improved sensitivity.[13] FDG-PET may identify disease involvement within normal-sized lymph nodes, or within extranodal sites, allowing for more accurate staging and confirmation of advanced stage. The intensity of FDG uptake, measured by the standardized uptake value (SUV), is highly heterogeneous in patients with follicular lymphoma. Earlier studies have suggested that higher SUV levels (>10) should increase suspicion for transformation to more aggressive histology and prompt a targeted biopsy.[14,15] Although it is noteworthy that data from the Gallium trial revealed that more than 65% of patients evaluated had a baseline maximum SUV level greater than 10 and did not correlate with risk of transformation,[16] it is important to remember that the SUV is calculated based on radioactivity concentration as measured by the PET scanner, the decay-corrected amount of injected FDG as well as the weight of the patient, and as a result is subject to significant variability because of physical and biological sources of error, inconsistent or nonoptimized image acquisition, processing, and analysis.[17,18]

An additional FDG-PET parameter that may have value at baseline in patients with FL is the total-body metabolic tumor volume (TMTV). Calculation of TMTV, made possible by improved algorithms and automation in recent years, evaluates the total volume of FDG-avid disease by drawing around 3-dimensional regions of interest using computer software.[19] In a retrospective analysis of 3 large clinical trials, investigators identified that the 29% of patients with pretreatment TMTV greater than 510 cm^3 had significantly inferior outcomes, and 5-year progression-free survival (PFS) estimates of only 32.7%, compared with 65.1% for those with lower TMTV.[19] Although this analysis has limitations (relatively small number of patients and the use of different PET scanners with associated potential for interscanner variability), it further highlights the potential role for baseline PET assessment in terms of prognostication and treatment selection.[2,13] An overview of recommended staging is presented in **Table 2**.

INITIAL TREATMENT OF HIGH TUMOR BURDEN FOLLICULAR LYMPHOMA: THE CHOICES

Once a patient has been identified as having high tumor burden disease, treatment selection should be individualized based on patient comorbidities, preferences, or concern for underlying transformation. Currently, the combination of an anti-CD20 monoclonal antibody with chemotherapy remains the standard of care. Common chemotherapy regimens used in this setting include those that spare the use of anthracycline for improved tolerability, either bendamustine or cyclophosphamide, vincristine, and prednisone (CVP), versus the upfront inclusion of doxorubicin using CHOP (cyclophosphamide, doxorubicin, vincristine, and prednisone).[20–23] More recently, a chemotherapy-"sparing" regimen using lenalidomide and rituximab upfront has also

Table 2	
Recommended staging of new patients with follicular lymphoma	
History	B symptoms (absence/presence of fevers to >101°F [38.3°C], drenching night sweats, or unexplained weight loss ≥ 10% of body mass within 6 mo)
	Significant pruritus
	Fatigue, change in performance status (ECOG)
	Early satiety, Left Upper Quadrant discomfort
	Dyspnea, increased abdominal girth
Physical examination	Peripheral lymphadenopathy
	Splenomegaly[a]
	Hepatomegaly
	Pleural effusions
	Ascites
Laboratory testing	Complete blood count and differential
	Immunophenotyping if unusual cells identified on peripheral blood smear or elevated absolute lymphocyte count
	Electrolyte panel
	Renal and liver function tests
	LDH and B2M
	Uric acid
	Serology: Hepatitis B, C, and human immunodeficiency virus
	Optional: serum protein electrophoresis & immunofixation
	Pregnancy testing in women of childbearing age
Imaging	CT neck, chest, abdomen, and pelvis
	Recommended: FDG-PET
Bone marrow	Aspirate & biopsy
	Optional: immunophenotyping, polymerase chain reaction or fluorescence in situ hybridization for BCL2 rearrangement
Consider	Cardiac assessment[b]

[a] More recent classification suggests enlarged if >13 cm in craniocaudal dimension.[13]
[b] If considering anthracyclines.

Data from Cheson, B.D., et al., Recommendations for initial evaluation, staging, and response assessment of Hodgkin and non-Hodgkin lymphoma: the Lugano classification. J Clin Oncol, 2014. **32**(27): p. 3059-68.

been evaluated (see later discussion).[24] Finally, single-agent rituximab may be an option for some patients if there is a contraindication for chemotherapy. A long-term follow-up analysis of trials involving rituximab alone, or in combination with interferon, demonstrates that while the duration of response is short in most patients (median time to treatment failure, 1.5 years), there is a small proportion that can experience prolonged disease control, with 30% still not requiring treatment at approximately 10 years of follow-up.[25] Similar results were reported in an updated analysis of the Swiss Group for Clinical Cancer Research trial of single-agent rituximab (which enrolled both treatment-naïve and chemotherapy-exposed patients) with median event-free estimates ranging from 1 to 2 years depending on whether patients received a prolonged or abbreviated rituximab schedule, and 27% of the prolonged schedule group were still without an event at 8 years.[26]

IS THERE AN OPTIMAL FRONTLINE CHEMOTHERAPY?

In the pre–rituximab era, chemotherapy regimens used to treat high tumor burden FL included chlorambucil, CVP, CHOP, and fludarabine-based regimens, such as fludarabine and mitoxantrone (FM), with no firm consensus for 1 regimen over another. Several randomized phase 3 studies subsequently demonstrated a significant improvement in outcome, including better overall survival (OS) with the addition of the anti-CD20 monoclonal antibody rituximab to various chemotherapy backbones.[27–29] As a result, immunochemotherapy became the standard of care for initial therapy for high tumor burden FL, but the optimal chemotherapy backbone remained controversial. The FOLL05 randomized trial compared the R-CHOP (rituximab plus cyclophosphamide, doxorubicin, vincristine, and prednisone), R-CVP (rituximab plus cyclophosphamide, vincristine, and prednisone), and R-FM (rituximab plus fludarabine and mitoxantrone) regimens, demonstrating an advantage for R-CHOP over R-CVP in terms of PFS, and excess toxicity associated with R-FM.[20,30] Importantly, despite mature follow-up, no difference in OS was observed between any of these regimens.[20] This finding was corroborated within a smaller randomized trial comparing R-CHOP with R-CVP.[31] An analysis of the National LymphoCare Study, adjusting for clinical risk factors, also failed to demonstrate a survival advantage associated with any particular chemotherapy regimen, including the use of frontline R-CHOP.[32]

After studies in the relapsed setting demonstrated notable efficacy, the bifunctional alkylator bendamustine was evaluated in combination with rituximab (BR) in the upfront setting in high tumor burden FL.[22,23,33] The StiL Trial compared BR to R-CHOP in patients with advanced-stage FL meeting GELF criteria and demonstrated significant benefit in favor of BR with a 39% reduction in PFS (hazard ratio [HR] 0.61; 95% confidence interval [CI]: 0.42–0.87; $P = .0072$). This benefit was found to be independent of age, LDH, and other baseline risk factors (including the FLIPI score). Ten-year follow-up has confirmed the long-term benefit of BR over R-CHOP in patients with indolent histology with the time-to-treatment failure almost doubled compared with R-CHOP.[21] In addition, lower rates of grade 3 to 4 hematological toxicity, alopecia, stomatitis, and infections were seen for the BR-treated patients.

The BRIGHT trial also evaluated BR induction in patients with indolent lymphomas, most of whom had FL grade 1 to 2, and similar to StiL, enrolled other histologies, such as mantle cell lymphoma. The objective of this study was to determine whether BR was noninferior (NI) to a "standard" comparator: R-CVP or R-CHOP. The trial met its primary endpoint because BR was demonstrated to be NI, with complete response (CR) rates of 31% versus 25% in the standard arm (CR rate ratio 1.26; $P = .0225$ for NI). Overall response rates (ORR) were also in favor of BR at 97% versus 91%, respectively. Although this trial was not intended to assess time-to-event endpoints, these were subsequently published and were uniformly in favor of BR compared with R-CHOP/R-CVP, with the strongest trends observed compared with those receiving R-CVP.[34] Extended follow-up of both the StiL and the BRIGHT trials has not demonstrated any difference in OS between BR and R-CHOP.[21,23,34]

Regardless of the underlying backbone chosen, patients with FL can expect excellent outcomes in the modern era of immunochemotherapy, with OS estimates of 80% at 10 years.[20,35] However, approximately 15% to 20% of patients will experience early progression, variably defined as progression within 2 years of diagnosis or initiation of therapy, the Progression of Disease (POD) 24 or event-free survival (EFS) 24 population.[36–39] These patients represent a higher-risk population with poorer outcomes, which is discussed in detail in a separate article in this series.

In the absence of early treatment failure or the development of transformation to a more aggressive histology, patients with follicular lymphoma treated with immunochemotherapy can expect excellent outcomes with reported event-free estimates of 75% to 87% at 2 years in population-based analyses,[36,38,40] and with an OS comparable to the general population.[41,42] Given the apparent improvement in PFS when compared with both R-CVP and R-CHOP, and the favorable safety profile allowing safe delivery to older patients or those with impaired cardiac or renal function, BR has become the preferred initial treatment of high tumor burden FL at many centers.[43,44] In addition, upfront BR spares the use of an anthracycline, which may be required at a later date in the event of histologic transformation, the risk of which appears unchanged despite the introduction of bendamustine with reported incidence of approximately 2% to 3% per year.[36,45–47]

It should be noted that a recent post hoc analysis of the Gallium trial, discussed in greater detail in later discussion, which was not designed to compare outcomes between the different chemotherapy backbones, demonstrated an increased incidence of grade 3 to 5 infections in patients receiving bendamustine.[48] In addition, especially in patients older than 70 years of age, a greater number of fatal adverse events (AE) were seen, compared with those who received CHOP or CVP. An increased proportion of fatal AEs had not been reported in prior trials involving BR and may in part be due to differences in patient risk profiles between the arms or the use of maintenance therapy within the Gallium trial.[44,49] Nonetheless, the possibility of delayed toxicities, including infection with the use of bendamustine, should be acknowledged, and patients should be monitored accordingly.

SPECIAL CONSIDERATIONS: GRADE 3A AND OCCULT TRANSFORMATION

Approximately 15% of patients with FL present with grade 3A disease, which has been associated with more proliferative disease, inferior outcomes, and increased risk of transformation.[47,50–52] Historically, the use of anthracycline-based therapy in patients with FL grade 3A demonstrated a plateau on the survival curve in some, but not all, retrospective series, which fueled controversy regarding optimal management.[53,54] Unfortunately, these patients have been excluded from most prospective trials, including StiL and BRIGHT, and therefore, randomized phase 3 evidence in this setting is lacking. Nonetheless, a recent retrospective analysis of 132 treatment-naïve patients with FL grade 3A with mature follow-up suggested that BR induction in this population achieved comparable response rates to R-CHOP, with improved PFS (median 15 vs 11.7 years, respectively, $P = .03$) and was associated with less toxicity, in line with the randomized prospective studies.[55] The investigators concluded that BR is a valid option for patients with FL grade 3A. Although prospective data are lacking, it would seem reasonable to consider BR for these patients in the absence of more aggressive, transformed disease.

In the absence of documented transformation, patients perceived to have an increased risk of occult transformation based on clinical, radiological, or laboratory findings may be best treated with anthracycline-based therapy to avoid the risk of undertreating aggressive histology disease.[15,46,56] A retrospective review of patients with follicular lymphoma treated with BR in British Columbia demonstrated that most early treatment failures after BR induction have evidence of transformed disease, suggesting that some may have harbored occult transformation at the time of initial treatment.[36] The pursuit of diagnostic tissue to confirm the presence of transformation should be attempted whenever possible. However, biopsy confirmation is not always feasible, and risk of a false negative biopsy can be high. In this instance, treatment decisions should be guided by a compilation of clinical factors, because patients with clinically presumed transformation have been shown to have similar outcomes to patients with pathologically confirmed transformation.[46] Established clinical parameters suggesting the occurrence of transformation include the presence of at least one of the following: sudden increase in LDH to twice the upper limit of normal; rapid discordant localized nodal growth detected clinically or by imaging studies; involvement of unusual extranodal sites (eg, liver, bone, brain); B symptoms; or the development of hypercalcemia,[46,56] or, as mentioned previously, elevated SUVs on FDG-PET.[14,15]

THE ROLE OF ANTI-CD20 MONOCLONAL ANTIBODIES

The introduction of the anti-CD20 monoclonal antibody rituximab was the first therapeutic to improve OS in FL. The initial regulatory approval of rituximab in 1997 in FL was based on data from a pivotal phase 2 trial of rituximab monotherapy in 166 patients with relapsed or refractory low-grade non-Hodgkin lymphoma.[57] There followed a series of trials performed in the front-line and relapsed settings, given as a monotherapy or in combination with various chemotherapy backbones, demonstrating its substantial clinical benefits: improvements in response rates and survival estimates without significant increase in toxicity.[27–29,58–61] More recently, the fully humanized glycoengineered anti-CD20 monoclonal antibody obinutuzumab was developed, with structural differences aimed to improve its efficacy as demonstrated in preclinical models. The potential differences between these 2 anti-CD20 monoclonal antibodies have been reviewed extensively elsewhere and are beyond the scope of this article.[62] After encouraging early-phase results in the relapsed and refractory setting, obinutuzumab was directly compared with rituximab in the upfront setting in the Gallium trial.[11] Gallium was one of the largest prospective trials ever performed in FL, enrolling more than 1200 patients meeting GELF criteria for high tumor burden who were randomized to receive either rituximab or obinutuzumab with chemotherapy as selected by the enrolling site, including CVP, CHOP, or bendamustine. Responding patients went on to receive 2 additional years of the assigned monoclonal antibody as maintenance.

After a median follow-up time of just 34.5 months, a planned interim analysis reported a significant reduction in 3-year PFS for the obinutuzumab-chemotherapy arm that was statistically superior to rituximab-chemotherapy arm (80% vs 73%, respectively; $P = .001$). Interestingly, response rates were similar between the arms, but a subsequent subgroup analysis demonstrated an increased proportion of patients in the obinutuzumab arm achieved minimal residual disease response, suggesting the novel antibody was able to induce deeper levels of response.[63] Higher rates of infusion-related events and neutropenia were reported for the obinutuzumab-containing arm, but toxicities were generally manageable and did not result in treatment compromise or excess mortality.

An interesting exploratory analysis evaluated the risk of early progression according to antibody received.[51] In total, 155 of 1071 patients with greater than 24 months of follow-up experienced progressive disease or death from progression within 2 years of randomization (POD24), and similar to previous published reports, outcomes for these early progressors were significantly inferior to their reference counterparts, with an age-adjusted HR for OS of 12.2 (95% CI: 5.6%–26.5%).[38,39,62,64] The risk of an early disease progression event (POD24) was significantly reduced in the obinutuzumab arm, with a cumulative incidence rate of 10.1% versus 17.4% in the rituximab arm, corresponding to an average risk reduction of 46% (95% CI: 25%–61%; $P = .0003$). Reducing these early progression events may ultimately have a significant impact on outcome, and updated results with more mature follow-up are eagerly awaited.

The Gallium trial led to the registration and approval of obinutuzumab combined with chemotherapy for symptomatic advanced-stage FL. However, based on the marginal improvement in 3-year PFS and lack of OS benefit, along with the increased toxicity and added drug costs, the use of obinutuzumab in the front-line setting for FL has not been universally adopted, with some centers reserving its use for higher-risk patients.[44,49,65] Finally, the use of anti-CD20 monoclonal antibodies (either rituximab or obinutuzumab) as maintenance after induction in responding patients is a commonly used practice based on data from randomized trials and is reviewed in depth elsewhere in this series.[11,12]

THE PROS AND CONS OF LENALIDOMIDE-RITUXIMAB

Given the excellent outcomes that can now be expected in patients with FL, with 80% alive at 10 years after diagnosis, and the potential for both short- and long-term toxicity with chemotherapy-containing induction regimens, a "chemotherapy-free" alternative remains desirable and was recently evaluated in a prospective trial.[24] In the RELEVANCE trial, patients with previously untreated FL meeting GELF criteria were randomized to either R^2 or R-chemo (investigators choice of BR, R-CHOP, or R-CVP).[24] Both cohorts were treated over a total of 120 weeks, as outlined in **Fig. 1**. All R^2 patients were treated with lenalidomide for a total of 18 cycles, whereas R-chemo was administered as standard (depending on the regimen) for 6 to 8 cycles. Both cohorts received rituximab maintenance (see **Fig. 1**).

Designed as a superiority study, results demonstrated no improvement in PFS for R^2 over R-chemo. Although this trial failed to meet its primary endpoint, with a median follow-up time of 37.9 months, a striking similarity in outcomes was observed for PFS (3-year estimates of 77% vs 78% for R^2 vs R-chemo) and OS (94% in both arms). On exploratory subgroup analysis, no subgroup was identified that appeared to preferentially benefit or exhibit worse outcomes with R^2. The overall rates of grade 3 to 5 adverse events were similar across both cohorts (65% R^2 vs 68% R-chemo), although the toxicity profiles were different. R-chemo was associated with more grade 3 to 4 neutropenia (50% R-chemo vs 32% R^2), whereas grade 3 to 4 cutaneous reactions were higher in the R^2 group (7% vs 1%). Infections of any grade (12% vs 5%) and grade 3 to 4 (4% vs 2%) were also higher in the R-chemo compared with the R^2 arm.

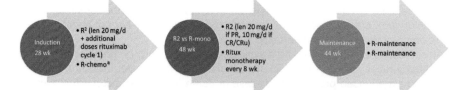

Fig. 1. Treatment schedule RELEVANCE trial. [a] R-chemo arms: R-CHOP: rituximab 375 mg/m² intravenous (IV) day 1, cyclophosphamide 750 mg/m² IV day 1, doxorubicin 50 mg/m² IV day 1, vincristine 1.4 mg/m² IV day 1, and prednisone 100 mg/d (orally days 1–5) for six 21-day cycles followed by two 21-day cycles of rituximab 375 mg/m², and 7 weeks later, responding patients continued with rituximab 375 mg/m² every 8 weeks for 12 cycles. BR: rituximab 375 mg/m² IV day 1 and bendamustine 90 mg/m² IV day 1 to 2 were given for six 28-day cycles; 8 weeks later, responding patients continued with rituximab 375 mg/m² every 8 weeks for 12 cycles. R-CVP: rituximab 375 mg/m² IV day 1, cyclophosphamide 750 mg/m² IV day 1, vincristine 1.4 mg/m² IV day 1, and prednisone 40 mg/d orally days 1 to 5 were given for eight 21-day cycles; 7 weeks later, responding patients continued with rituximab 375 mg/m² every 8 weeks for 12 cycles. CRu, complete response unconfirmed; PR, partial response.

Based on this trial, R^2 appears to result in comparable outcomes to R-chemo, albeit with a prolonged induction schedule and with likely higher cost. A shorter R^2 duration of therapy has been evaluated, given for just 18 weeks, with median PFS of 5 years for the combination and median time to next treatment still not reached at 4 years of follow-up.[66] In addition, the combination of lenalidomide with obinutuzumab has been recently reported with very impressive outcomes albeit with limited follow-up of just 22 months. In this high tumor burden population, reported 2-year PFS was 96%, ORR was 98%, and 92% of patients achieved a CR at the first response assessment (cycle 4, day 1).[67] More mature follow-up data from this study are eagerly awaited.

At the current time, for those patients in whom immunochemotherapy is contraindicated or those who prefer a "chemotherapy-free" approach, R^2 would appear to be a reasonable option, although the available data to date remain immature and the potential for longer term side effects as well as the optimal duration and sequencing of R^2 remains uncertain.

POST-THERAPY SURVEILLANCE: CAN PATIENTS EVER BE DISCHARGED?

Although patients treated in the modern era have excellent outcomes and can achieve long-term disease control following frontline therapy, FL remains incurable, and most patients will inevitably relapse. The frequency of post-treatment surveillance is variable in clinical practice, but published recommendations suggest an initial schedule of every 3 to 6 months as determined by pretreatment risk factors, the depth of response, and ongoing management strategy.[2,13] Predicting patients at increased risk of early progression remains challenging, but recent data have demonstrated potential utility of post-induction FDG-PET scan results that may serve to identify patients who warrant closer initial surveillance.[68,69] Certainly, the initial 24 months are the most crucial period for surveillance, because patients who demonstrate evidence of early progression (the POD24/EFS24 population) are at greatest risk for inferior survival.[36,38,39,64,70,71] The biology and management of this high-risk population are discussed in greater depth in a separate article in this series. The subset of patients (70%–87%) that reaches the 2-year landmark without experiencing relapse can expect very favorable outcomes with OS estimates ranging from 90% at 5 years to 80% at 10 years.[38,39,51,71] However, because these patients at very low risk for relapse cannot readily be identified, active surveillance within a specialty practice remains prudent.

Current guidelines suggest that patients at low risk of recurrence beyond the 2-year mark should be seen biannually to annually, with a focused history, physical examination, and laboratory tests, including a complete blood count, LDH level, and basic metabolic panel.[2,13] Given supportive evidence that there is little gained by routine surveillance imaging, updated recommendations have largely discouraged this practice.[13,72] Exceptions may include higher-risk patients such as those with positive post-treatment FDG-PET scans, or patients who harbor disease exclusively in sites that are difficult to monitor by physical examination alone. In such patients, the "judicious use" of surveillance imaging can be considered.[13]

SUMMARY

In the current era, patients with FL despite having high tumor burden can expect excellent outcomes following initial therapy. In the absence of early treatment failure or histologic transformation, the vast majority (>80%) will still be alive at 10 years, and many may not require further treatment within their lifetime. Upfront immunochemotherapy remains the standard of care, following improvements in both PFS and OS seen with the introduction of anti-CD20 monoclonal antibodies, and selection of initial chemotherapy backbone should be tailored to patient and disease characteristics, although BR has largely become the preferred regimen in many centers. In view of the comparable outcomes observed with lenalidomide and rituximab, this regimen may be an alternative for patients with a contraindication to standard chemotherapy. Vigilance for early treatment failure (within 2 years) and the ongoing risk of histologic transformation is needed, because the ability to identify and optimally manage these high-risk patients remains a significant unmet need and the subject of ongoing research.

DISCLOSURE

Dr C.L. Freeman reports honoraria from Seattle Genetics, Janssen, Amgen, Celgene, Sanofi, and Abbvie, and research funding from Roche and Teva. Dr L.H. Sehn reports consultancy fees, honoraria from Karyopharm; consultancy fees from Abbvie, Apobiologix, Astra-Zeneca, Acerta, Roche/Genentech, Gilead, Seattle Genetics, Amgen, Celgene, Morphosys, Kite, TG Therapeutics, Merck, Lundbeck, Janssen, Karyopharm, Verastem; and research funding from Roche/Genentech.

REFERENCES

1. Nooka AK, Nabhan C, Zhou X, et al. Examination of the follicular lymphoma international prognostic index (FLIPI) in the National LymphoCare study (NLCS): a prospective US patient cohort treated predominantly in community practices 2013;24(2):441–8.
2. Dreyling M, Ghielmini M, Rule S, et al. Newly diagnosed and relapsed follicular lymphoma: ESMO Clinical Practice Guidelines for diagnosis, treatment and follow-up. Ann Oncol 2016;27(suppl 5):v83–90.
3. Solal-Celigny P, Lepage E, Brousse N, et al. Doxorubicin-containing regimen with or without interferon alfa-2b for advanced follicular lymphomas: final analysis of survival and toxicity in the Groupe d'Etude des Lymphomes Folliculaires 86 Trial. J Clin Oncol 1998;16(7):2332–8.
4. Brice P, Bastion Y, Lepage E, et al. Comparison in low-tumor-burden follicular lymphomas between an initial no-treatment policy, prednimustine, or interferon alfa: a randomized study from the Groupe d'Etude des Lymphomes Folliculaires. Groupe d'Etude des Lymphomes de l'Adulte. J Clin Oncol 1997;15(3):1110–7.
5. Solal-Celigny P, Roy P, Colombat P, et al. Follicular lymphoma international prognostic index. Blood 2004;104(5):1258–65.
6. Federico M, Bellei M, Marcheselli L, et al. Follicular lymphoma international prognostic index 2: a new prognostic index for follicular lymphoma developed by the international follicular lymphoma prognostic factor project. J Clin Oncol 2009; 27(27):4555–62.
7. Bachy E, Maurer MJ, Habermann TM, et al. A simplified scoring system in de novo follicular lymphoma treated initially with immunochemotherapy. Blood 2018;132(1):49–58.
8. Montoto S, Lopez-Guillermo A, Altes A, et al. Predictive value of Follicular Lymphoma International Prognostic Index (FLIPI) in patients with follicular lymphoma at first progression. Ann Oncol 2004;15(10):1484–9.
9. Buske C, Hoster E, Dreyling M, et al. The Follicular Lymphoma International Prognostic Index (FLIPI) separates high-risk from intermediate- or low-risk patients with advanced-stage follicular lymphoma treated front-line with rituximab and

the combination of cyclophosphamide, doxorubicin, vincristine, and prednisone (R-CHOP) with respect to treatment outcome. Blood 2006;108(5):1504–8.

10. Ardeshna K, Smith P, Norton A, et al. Long-term effect of a watch and wait policy versus immediate systemic treatment for asymptomatic advanced-stage non-Hodgkin lymphoma: a randomised controlled trial. The Lancet 2003;362(9383): 516–22.

11. Marcus R, Davies A, Ando K, et al. Obinutuzumab for the first-line treatment of follicular lymphoma. N Engl J Med 2017;377(14):1331–44.

12. Salles G, Seymour JF, Offner F, et al. Rituximab maintenance for 2 years in patients with high tumour burden follicular lymphoma responding to rituximab plus chemotherapy (PRIMA): a phase 3, randomised controlled trial. Lancet 2011;377(9759):42–51.

13. Cheson BD, Fisher RI, Barrington SF, et al. Recommendations for initial evaluation, staging, and response assessment of Hodgkin and non-Hodgkin lymphoma: the Lugano classification. J Clin Oncol 2014;32(27):3059–68.

14. Schoder H, Noy A, Gonen M, et al. Intensity of 18fluorodeoxyglucose uptake in positron emission tomography distinguishes between indolent and aggressive non-Hodgkin's lymphoma. J Clin Oncol 2005;23(21):4643–51.

15. Noy A, Schoder H, Gonen M, et al. The majority of transformed lymphomas have high standardized uptake values (SUVs) on positron emission tomography (PET) scanning similar to diffuse large B-cell lymphoma (DLBCL). Ann Oncol 2009; 20(3):508–12.

16. Mir F, Barrington SF, Meignan M, et al. Baseline suvmax did not predict histological transformation from follicular lymphoma to aggressive lymphoma in the phase III GALLIUM study. Blood 2018;132(Suppl 1):4160.

17. Kinahan PE, Fletcher JW. Positron emission tomography-computed tomography standardized uptake values in clinical practice and assessing response to therapy. Semin Ultrasound CT MR 2010;31(6):496–505.

18. Boellaard R, Krak NC, Hoekstra OS, et al. Effects of noise, image resolution, and ROI definition on the accuracy of standard uptake values: a simulation study. J Nucl Med 2004;45(9):1519–27.

19. Meignan M, Cottereau AS, Versari A, et al. Baseline metabolic tumor volume predicts outcome in high–tumor-burden follicular lymphoma: a pooled analysis of three multicenter studies. Journal of Clinical Oncology 2016;34(30):3618–26.

20. Luminari S, Ferrari A, Manni M, et al. Long-term results of the FOLL05 trial comparing R-CVP versus R-CHOP versus R-FM for the initial treatment of patients with advanced-stage symptomatic follicular lymphoma. Journal of Clinical Oncology 2018;36(7):689–96.

21. Rummel MJ, Maschmeyer G, Ganser A, et al. Bendamustine plus rituximab (B-R) versus CHOP plus rituximab (CHOP-R) as first-line treatment in patients with indolent lymphomas: nine-year updated results from the StiL NHL1 study. Journal of Clinical Oncology 2017;35(15_suppl):7501.

22. Rummel MJ, Niederle N, Maschmeyer G, et al. Bendamustine plus rituximab versus CHOP plus rituximab as first-line treatment for patients with indolent and mantle-cell lymphomas: an open-label, multicentre, randomised, phase 3 non-inferiority trial. Lancet 2013;381(9873):1203–10.

23. Flinn IW, van der Jagt R, Kahl BS, et al. Randomized trial of bendamustine-rituximab or R-CHOP/R-CVP in first-line treatment of indolent NHL or MCL: the BRIGHT study. Blood 2014;123(19):2944–52.

24. Morschhauser F, Fowler NH, Feugier P, et al. Rituximab plus lenalidomide in advanced untreated follicular lymphoma. New England Journal of Medicine 2018;379(10):934–47.

25. Lockmer S, Østenstad B, Hagberg H, et al. Chemotherapy-free initial treatment of advanced indolent lymphoma has durable effect with low toxicity: results from two nordic lymphoma group trials with more than 10 years of follow-up. Journal of Clinical Oncology 2018;36(33):3315–23.

26. Martinelli G, Schmitz SF, Utiger U, et al. Long-term follow-up of patients with follicular lymphoma receiving single-agent rituximab at two different schedules in trial SAKK 35/98. J Clin Oncol 2010;28(29):4480–4.

27. Marcus R, Imrie K, Solal-Celigny P, et al. Phase III study of R-CVP compared with cyclophosphamide, vincristine, and prednisone alone in patients with previously untreated advanced follicular lymphoma. Journal of Clinical Oncology 2008; 26(28):4579–86.

28. Hiddemann W, Kneba M, Dreyling M, et al. Frontline therapy with rituximab added to the combination of cyclophosphamide, doxorubicin, vincristine, and prednisone (CHOP) significantly improves the outcome for patients with advanced-stage follicular lymphoma compared with therapy with CHOP alone: results of a prospective randomized study of the German Low-Grade Lymphoma Study Group. Blood 2005;106(12):3725–32.

29. Herold M, Haas A, Srock S, et al. Rituximab added to first-line mitoxantrone, chlorambucil, and prednisolone chemotherapy followed by interferon maintenance prolongs survival in patients with advanced follicular lymphoma: an East German Study Group Hematology and Oncology Study. J Clin Oncol 2007; 25(15):1986–92.

30. Federico M, Luminari S, Dondi A, et al. R-CVP versus R-CHOP versus R-FM for the initial treatment of patients with advanced-stage follicular lymphoma: results of the FOLL05 trial conducted by the Fondazione Italiana Linfomi 2013;31(12): 1506–13.

31. Walewski J, Paszkiewicz-Kozik E, Michalski W, et al. First-line R-CVP versus R-CHOP induction immunochemotherapy for indolent lymphoma with rituximab maintenance. A multicentre, phase III randomized study by the Polish Lymphoma Research Group PLRG4. Br J Haematol 2019.

32. Nastoupil LJ, Sinha R, Byrtek M, et al. Comparison of the effectiveness of frontline chemoimmunotherapy regimens for follicular lymphoma used in the United States. Leuk Lymphoma 2015;56(5):1295–302.

33. Cheson BD, Rummel MJ. Bendamustine: rebirth of an old drug. J Clin Oncol 2009;27(9):1492–501.

34. Flinn IW, Van Der Jagt R, Kahl B, et al. First-line treatment of patients with indolent Non-Hodgkin Lymphoma or Mantle-Cell Lymphoma with Bendamustine Plus Rituximab Versus R-CHOP or R-CVP: results of the BRIGHT 5-year follow-up study. Journal of Clinical Oncology 2019;37(12):984–91.

35. Salles GA, Seymour JF, Feugier P, et al. Long term follow-up of the PRIMA study: half of patients receiving rituximab maintenance remain progression free at 10 years. Blood 2017;130(Suppl 1):486.

36. Freeman CL, Kridel R, Moccia AA, et al. Early progression after bendamustine-rituximab is associated with high risk of transformation in advanced stage follicular lymphoma. Blood 2019;134(9):761–4.

37. Maurer MJ, Ghesquieres H, Jais JP, et al. Event-free survival at 24 months is a robust end point for disease-related outcome in diffuse large B-cell lymphoma treated with immunochemotherapy. J Clin Oncol 2014;32(10):1066–73.

38. Maurer MJ, Jakopsen LH, Habermann TM, et al. Outcomes after early transformation (tPOD24) VS. early follicular lymphoma progression (fPOD24) in follicular lymphoma treated with frontline immunochemotherapy. Hematol Oncol 2019;37: 231–2.

39. Casulo C, Byrtek M, Dawson KL, et al. Early relapse of follicular lymphoma after rituximab plus cyclophosphamide, doxorubicin, vincristine, and prednisone defines patients at high risk for death: an analysis from the national lymphocare study. Journal of Clinical Oncology 2015;33(23):2516–22.

40. Mondello P, Steiner N, Willenbacher W, et al. Bendamustine plus rituximab versus R-CHOP as first-line treatment for patients with indolent non-Hodgkin's lymphoma: evidence from a multicenter, retrospective study. Ann Hematol 2016; 95(7):1107–14.

41. Magnano L, Alonso-Alvarez S, Alcoceba M, et al. Life expectancy of follicular lymphoma patients in complete response at 30 months is similar to that of the Spanish general population. Br J Haematol 2019;185(3):480–91.

42. Provencio M, Royuela A, Torrente M, et al. Prognostic value of event-free survival at 12 and 24 months and long-term mortality for non-Hodgkin follicular lymphoma patients: a study report from the Spanish Lymphoma Oncology Group. Cancer 2017;123(19):3709–16.

43. Storti S, Spina M, Pesce EA, et al. Rituximab plus bendamustine as front-line treatment in frail elderly (>70 years) patients with diffuse large B-cell non-Hodgkin lymphoma: a phase II multicenter study of the Fondazione Italiana Linfomi. Haematologica 2018;103(8):1345–50.

44. Friedberg JW. Progress in advanced-stage follicular lymphoma. Journal of Clinical Oncology 2018;36(23):2363–5.

45. Fischer T, Zing NPC, Chiattone CS, et al. Transformed follicular lymphoma. Ann Hematol 2018;97(1):17–29.

46. Al-Tourah AJ, Gill KK, Chhanabhai M, et al. Population-based analysis of incidence and outcome of transformed non-Hodgkin's lymphoma. J Clin Oncol 2008;26(32):5165–9.

47. Montoto S, Davies AJ, Matthews J, et al. Risk and clinical implications of transformation of follicular lymphoma to diffuse large B-cell lymphoma 2007;25(17): 2426–33.

48. Hiddemann W, Barbui AM, Canales MA, et al. Immunochemotherapy with obinutuzumab or rituximab for previously untreated follicular lymphoma in the GALLIUM study: influence of chemotherapy on efficacy and safety. Journal of Clinical Oncology 2018;36(23):2395–404.

49. Armitage JO, Longo DL. Which anti-CD20 antibody is better in follicular lymphoma? New England Journal of Medicine 2017;377(14):1389–90.

50. Sarkozy C, Trneny M, Xerri L, et al. Risk factors and outcomes for patients with follicular lymphoma who had histologic transformation after response to first-line immunochemotherapy in the PRIMA trial. J Clin Oncol 2016;34(22):2575–82.

51. Seymour JF, Marcus R, Davies A, et al. Association of early disease progression and very poor survival in the GALLIUM study in follicular lymphoma: benefit of obinutuzumab in reducing the rate of early progression. Haematologica 2019; 104(6):1202–8.

52. Winter AM, Nastoupil LJ, Becnel MR, et al. Outcomes of follicular lymphoma patients treated with frontline bendamustine and rituximab: impact of histologic grade and early progression on overall survival. Blood 2018;132(Suppl 1):4146.

53. Shustik J, Quinn M, Connors JM, et al. Follicular non-Hodgkin lymphoma grades 3A and 3B have a similar outcome and appear incurable with anthracycline-based therapy. Ann Oncol 2011;22(5):1164–9.
54. Ganti AK, Weisenburger DD, Smith LM, et al. Patients with grade 3 follicular lymphoma have prolonged relapse-free survival following anthracycline-based chemotherapy: the Nebraska Lymphoma Study Group Experience. Ann Oncol 2006;17(6):920–7.
55. Mondello P, Steiner N, Willenbacher W, et al. Bendamustine plus rituximab versus R-CHOP as first-line treatment for patients with follicular lymphoma Grade 3A: evidence from a multicenter, retrospective study. Oncologist 2018;23(4):454–60.
56. Link BK, Maurer MJ, Nowakowski GS, et al. Rates and outcomes of follicular lymphoma transformation in the immunochemotherapy era: a report from the University of Iowa/Mayo Clinic Specialized Program of Research Excellence Molecular Epidemiology Resource. Journal of Clinical Oncology 2013;31(26):3272–8.
57. McLaughlin P, Grillo-Lopez AJ, Link BK, et al. Rituximab chimeric anti-CD20 monoclonal antibody therapy for relapsed indolent lymphoma: half of patients respond to a four-dose treatment program. J Clin Oncol 1998;16(8):2825–33.
58. Czuczman MS, Weaver R, Alkuzweny B, et al. Prolonged clinical and molecular remission in patients with low-grade or follicular Non-Hodgkin's Lymphoma treated with Rituximab Plus CHOP chemotherapy: 9-year follow-up. Journal of Clinical Oncology 2004;22(23):4711–6.
59. Ardeshna KM, Qian W, Smith P, et al. Rituximab versus a watch-and-wait approach in patients with advanced-stage, asymptomatic, non-bulky follicular lymphoma: an open-label randomised phase 3 trial. Lancet Oncol 2014;15(4):424–35.
60. Forstpointner R, Dreyling M, Repp R, et al. The addition of rituximab to a combination of fludarabine, cyclophosphamide, mitoxantrone (FCM) significantly increases the response rate and prolongs survival as compared with FCM alone in patients with relapsed and refractory follicular and mantle cell lymphomas: results of a prospective randomized study of the German Low-Grade Lymphoma Study Group. Blood 2004;104(10):3064–71.
61. van Oers MH, Klasa R, Marcus RE, et al. Rituximab maintenance improves clinical outcome of relapsed/resistant follicular non-Hodgkin lymphoma in patients both with and without rituximab during induction: results of a prospective randomized phase 3 intergroup trial. Blood 2006;108(10):3295–301.
62. Freeman CL, Sehn LH. A tale of two antibodies: obinutuzumab versus rituximab. Br J Haematol 2018;182(1):29–45.
63. Pott C, Hoster E, Kehden B, et al. Minimal residual disease in patients with follicular lymphoma treated with obinutuzumab or rituximab as first-line induction immunochemotherapy and maintenance in the phase 3 GALLIUM study. Blood 2016;128(22):613.
64. Maurer MJ, Bachy E, Ghesquieres H, et al. Early event status informs subsequent outcome in newly diagnosed follicular lymphoma. Am J Hematol 2016;91(11):1096–101.
65. NICE Technology appraisal guidance: Obinutuzumab for untreated advanced follicular lymphoma. 2018. Available at: www.nice.org.uk/guidance/ta513. Accessed April 14, 2020.
66. Zucca E, Rondeau S, Vanazzi A, et al. Short regimen of rituximab plus lenalidomide in follicular lymphoma patients in need of first-line therapy. Blood 2019;134(4):353–62.

67. Nastoupil LJ, Westin JR, Hagemeister FB, et al. Results of a phase II study of obi-nutuzumab in combination with lenalidomide in previously untreated, high tumor burden follicular lymphoma (FL). Blood 2019;134(Supplement_1):125.
68. Trotman J, Luminari S, Boussetta S, et al. Prognostic value of PET-CT after first-line therapy in patients with follicular lymphoma: a pooled analysis of central scan review in three multicentre studies. The Lancet Haematology 2014;1(1): e17–27.
69. Dupuis J, Berriolo-Riedinger A, Julian A, et al. Impact of [(18)F]fluorodeoxyglu-cose positron emission tomography response evaluation in patients with high-tu-mor burden follicular lymphoma treated with immunochemotherapy: a prospective study from the Groupe d'Etudes des Lymphomes de l'Adulte and GOELAMS. J Clin Oncol 2012;30(35):4317–22.
70. Sarkozy C, Maurer MJ, Link BK, et al. Cause of death in follicular lymphoma in the first decade of the rituximab era: a pooled analysis of French and US cohorts. Journal of Clinical Oncology 2019;37(2):144–52.
71. Bachy E, Seymour JF, Feugier P, et al. Sustained progression-free survival benefit of rituximab maintenance in patients with follicular lymphoma: long-term results of the PRIMA study. Journal of Clinical Oncology 2019;37(31):2815–24.
72. Goldman ML, Kim C, Chen Z, et al. Surveillance imaging during first-remission in follicular lymphoma does not impact overall survival. Blood 2017;130(Suppl 1): 1501.

Antibody Therapy Maintenance in Follicular Lymphoma

Camille Golfier, MD, Gilles Salles, MD, PhD*

KEYWORDS

- Follicular lymphoma • Maintenance therapy • Rituximab • Anti-CD20 antibodies

KEY POINTS

- Patients with follicular lymphoma (FL) have a very high risk of disease recurrence, and options such as maintenance to prolong response after induction therapy might optimize their management.
- As evaluated in multiple randomized studies, rituximab maintenance (RM) therapy significantly delays the risk of disease progression in both low-tumor-burden and high-tumor-burden FL after induction therapy. However, the beneficial effect on overall survival in long-term follow-up remains debatable.
- The optimal RM schedule remains unknown, but rituximab administered every 2 months for 4 doses and every 2 or 3 months for 2 years seems to be the most commonly accepted scheme for patients responding to single-agent induction and immunochemotherapy induction, respectively.
- The main adverse events caused by rituximab maintenance include neutropenia and infections, which are manageable overall. In cases of unacceptable or recurrent toxicities during maintenance, discontinuation of treatment should be considered.

RATIONALE FOR ANTI-CD20–BASED MAINTENANCE TREATMENT

The introduction of rituximab to first-line and salvage therapies has significantly improved the prognosis of patients with follicular lymphoma (FL) during the last 2 decades. The median overall survival (OS) has been increased to 15 years or more.[1,2] However, FL, especially advanced-stage FL, is thought to remain incurable in most patients because of inevitable relapses. After the initial relapse, both the response

Hospices Civils de Lyon, Hôpital Lyon-Sud, Department of Hematology, Pierre-Bénite France and Université de Lyon, Université Claude Bernard, Faculté de Médecine Lyon-Sud, 165, chemin du Grand Revoyet, 69495 cedex, Oullins, France
* Corresponding author. Service d'Hématologie, Hôpital Lyon-Sud, 165, chemin du Grand Revoyet, Pierre Bénite Cedex 69495. France.
E-mail address: gilles.salles@chu-lyon.fr
Twitter: @gilles_salles (G.S.)

Hematol Oncol Clin N Am 34 (2020) 689–699
https://doi.org/10.1016/j.hoc.2020.02.005
0889-8588/20/© 2020 Elsevier Inc. All rights reserved.

hemonc.theclinics.com

rate and relapse-free survival decrease steadily, resulting in shrinking survival as subsequent disease progressions occur. Therefore, the main challenge of FL therapy seems to be more about extending the duration of the initial remission (ie, delaying relapses) without significantly increasing regimen toxicity than improving OS in this indolent disease.

The concept of maintenance therapy offering continued treatment to patients after successful induction therapy emerged as an effective option almost 20 years ago in an attempt to prevent the reemergence of disease. Because of the lack of long-term OS benefits and the significant toxicity observed, the use of cytotoxic agents (cyclophosphamide or chlorambucil) or interferon-alfa as maintenance therapy is no longer recommended.[3–5] Developing the use of anti–cluster of differentiation (CD) 20 monoclonal antibodies (MoAbs) for maintenance therapy in FL seemed relevant and appealing for several reasons. First, the pioneer anti-CD20 MoAb rituximab has proven efficacy as monotherapy in the relapse setting or as induction treatment in patients with FL, with limited acute toxicity and no major long-term or cumulative toxic effects. Moreover, administration modalities are simple, with an outpatient setting of particular importance for patients.

Regarding pharmacodynamics, a large body of evidence shows that rituximab induces FL cell death in vivo by different pathways, such as induction of apoptosis, complement-mediated cytolysis, and antibody-dependent cellular cytotoxicity.[6] The contribution of each of these mechanisms in mediating the clinical effects of the drug is still not well defined. In addition, the drug might also promote uptake and cross-presentation of lymphoma cell–derived peptides by antigen-presenting dendritic cells (DCs), induce maturation of DCs, and allow the generation of specific cytotoxic T lymphocytes.[7] It can hence be hypothesized that the so-called vaccinal effect (corresponding with the lymphoma-specific mediated T-cell response) could help offset the FL-induced inhibition of immune response and maintain a long-term pressure to control potential residual lymphoma cells.[8] It is also conceivable that rituximab maintenance (RM) may deplete the pool of FL precursors hidden in their niches[9] or of FL cancer repopulating cells that express the CD20 antigen (**Fig. 1**).

RITUXIMAB MAINTENANCE FOR LOW-TUMOR-BURDEN ADVANCED-STAGE FOLLICULAR LYMPHOMA

In 2002, Hainsworth and colleagues[10] showed that RM consisting of 4 weekly rituximab infusions administered every 6 months for 24 months improved the overall response rate (ORR) and especially complete response rate (CR) of 30% after standard (4 weekly infusions) single-agent rituximab induction (RI) treatment in patients with FL without causing additional toxicity. Median progression-free survival (PFS) was 34 months after RM versus 12 months after RI alone, a control median PFS observed in pivotal studies.[11]

The randomized phase III Swiss Group for Clinical Cancer Research (SAKK) 35/98 trial investigated RM (with a schedule of 1 infusion every 2 months for 4 infusions) after RI versus observation in 202 patients with FL, of whom 51 were newly diagnosed.[12,13] Compared with observation, RM prolonged median event-free survival (EFS) from 13 to 24 months (*P*<.001) after a median follow-up of 9.5 years. The best outcome was observed for previously untreated patients responding to RI (n = 38): EFS at 8 years was 45% in the RM arm versus 22% for the observation arm in this subgroup (*P*<.001). Although RM was not associated with additional toxicity, no difference was observed in terms of OS.

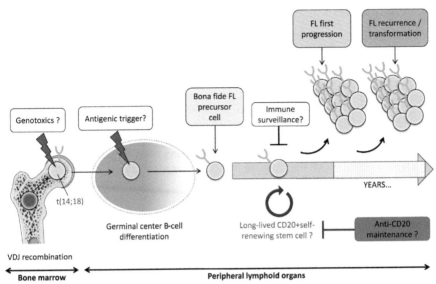

Fig. 1. Rationale for anti-CD20–based maintenance treatment. The t (14;18) (q32; q21) translocation is the genetic hallmark and early initiating event of FL. As a consequence, the *BCL2* gene comes under the control of the *IGH* enhancer, causing deregulated expression of the antiapoptotic BCL2 protein. B cells carrying t (14;18) and having transited through germinal centers may constitute potent premalignant FL cells that can further develop into true FL clonal precursor cells (CPCs). The repeated FL clinical appearance and manifestations of FL might be the consequence of the persistence and proliferation of these long-lived CD20+ self-renewing CPCs escaping from the immune surveillance system. The concept of anti-CD20 maintenance therapy may alter the pool or proliferation potential of these CD20+ CPCs and hence represent an effective option to prevent the reemergence of the disease. (*Data from* Roulland S, Navarro J-M, Grenot P, et al. Follicular lymphoma-like B cells in healthy individuals: a novel intermediate step in early lymphomagenesis. *J Exp Med.* 2006;203(11):2425-2431. https://doi.org/10.1084/jem. 20061292)

A large phase III trial evaluated the role of rituximab in delaying the need for treatment (chemotherapy or radiotherapy) in 379 newly diagnosed patients with FL.[14] All of them were asymptomatic and had advanced-stage FL with a low tumor burden. They were randomly assigned to watchful waiting (WW), RI alone (375 mg/m^2 every week for 4 weeks), or RI followed by RM with a schedule of 12 further infusions given every 2 months for 2 years. There was no significant difference in the time to start a new treatment between the RI and RM groups, but the RI arm had been prematurely closed in the study for slow accrual. Of note, at month 7, the quality of life (QoL) was significantly improved in the RM group, with more patients feeling in control of their disease and experiencing less anxiety about their diagnosis ($P = .007$). Compared with the RI arm, RM was associated with significantly better PFS (82% at 3 years) and better ORR at 25 months (84% vs 57%; $P = .001$), but there was no OS difference between the two groups.

Regarding the duration of maintenance, a long-term RM schedule (1 infusion every 2 months for 5 years) was assessed in the SAKK 35/03 trial against the initial RM schedule (4 infusions in 8 months). This prolonged maintenance did not show any improvement of EFS (main end point) or OS and was associated with significantly increased toxicity.[15]

MAINTENANCE THERAPY OR RETREATMENT?

Even though RM had been shown to improve the duration of remission and PFS in relapsed/refractory (R/R) patients with FL, Davis and colleagues[16] also observed that retreatment (4 weekly doses of rituximab) responders at the time of progression produced second remissions in 40% of patients, with a median duration of second responses reaching 18 months. Therefore, the question of whether RM could bring a relative benefit compared with rituximab retreatment (RR) at progression has arisen.

A first randomized phase II study allocated R/R patients responding to a previous standard RI to receive either RM (rituximab infusions every 6 months for 2 years) or RR (same schedule) at the time of lymphoma progression: PFS with RM was 31 months versus 13 months with RR.[17] However, the duration of disease control was similar between the study arms (31 and 35 months for RM and RR, respectively), as was the 3-year OS (72% and 68%, respectively).

In addition, the US-based RESORT (Rituximab Extended Schedule Or Retreatment) study randomized 289 newly diagnosed patients with low-burden FL responding after classic RI between RM and RR at the time of progression.[18] Patients assigned to RM received a single dose of rituximab every 3 months, whereas patients randomized in the RR arm were retreated with rituximab single agent (4 weekly infusions) at each disease progression, both until antibody treatment failure. Overall, the RR strategy provided a disease control comparable with that of the RM strategy. With a median follow-up of 4.5 years, there was no difference between the study arms in terms of the median time to treatment failure (3.9 vs 4.3 years, respectively; $P = .54$). There was a small advantage for RM regarding time to first cytotoxic therapy (3-year freedom from cytotoxic therapy 95% for RM vs 84% for RR; $P = .03$), but significantly more rituximab was required to achieve this benefit (4 doses for the RR group; 18 doses for the RM group). Although both RM and RR were well tolerated, RM was associated with significantly decreased serum immunoglobulin levels, and 1 patient died of progressive multifocal leukoencephalopathy (PML). Unlike the previously described UK trial comparing RM versus WW as first-line treatment of FL, no health-related QoL difference was observed in the RESORT study.

RITUXIMAB MAINTENANCE AFTER RITUXIMAB CHEMOTHERAPY

The European Organisation for Research and Treatment of Cancer (EORTC) 20981 phase III trial assessed the efficacy of RM in 334 randomized rituximab-naive R/R patients with FL who achieved a CR or partial response (PR) after receiving CHOP (cyclophosphamide, doxorubicin, vincristine, and prednisone) or CHOP plus rituximab (R-CHOP) as salvage therapy. After a median follow-up of 6 years, RM (375 mg/m^2 once every 3 months for 2 years) significantly improved median PFS compared with observation (3.7 years in the RM group vs 1.3 years in the WW group; hazard ratio [HR] = 0.55; $P<.001$). This benefit was observed independently of the chemotherapy treatment (CHOP vs R-CHOP) and across different FLIPI (Follicular Lymphoma International Prognostic Index) scores.[19,20] Of note, although the study was not powered to show an effect of RM on OS, 5-year OS rates (74% in the RM vs 64% in the observation arm; $P = .07$) indicated a trend favoring the use of maintenance. RM was well tolerated, with an increased incidence of grade 3 to 4 infections as the only significant adverse effects, which required only 4% of patients to discontinue RM. Likewise, Forstpointner and colleagues[21] observed a significant prolongation of median duration of response with RM (4 weekly doses given at month 3 and month 9 compared with observation) in 81 patients with R/R FL responding to salvage therapy (using a rituximab plus fludarabine–based combination: the median was not reached in the RM group vs 26 months for observation; $P = .035$). Side effects were similar in both arms.

Whether RM following different rituximab chemotherapy (R-chemo)–based regimens could improve outcomes in patients with advanced-stage high-tumor-burden FL treated as first-line therapy was the main question raised in the PRIMA (Primary Rituximab and Maintenance) trial conducted worldwide from 2004 to 2007.[22,23] A total of 1018 previously untreated patients achieving a CR or a PR after the R-chemo induction regimen (R-CHOP, R-CVP [rituximab, cyclophosphamide, vincristine, prednisone], or R-FCM [rituximab, fludarabine, cyclophosphamide, mitoxantrone]) were randomly assigned to RM or observation. Maintenance therapy consisted of 2 years of rituximab 375 mg/m^2 every 8 weeks. After a median follow-up of 9 years, the median PFS (primary end point) was 10.5 years in the RM arm versus 4.1 years in the observation group (HR, 0.61; 95% CI, 0.52–0.73; $P<.001$). Projected 10-year PFS was 51.1% in the RM arm and 35% in the observation arm. Patients in CR, CRu, or PR at the end of induction consistently benefited from RM. RM also provided a significant benefit compared with observation in terms of time to next lymphoma treatment, which was not reached in the RM arm but was 6.1 years in the control group ($P<.001$). Likewise, the time to next chemotherapy was not reached with RM but approached 9.3 years in the observation arm ($P<.001$). The PFS improvement associated with RM was independent of the induction R-chemo regimen or FLIPI score. No OS difference was seen in patients randomly assigned to both groups (HR = 1.04; 95% CI, 0.77–1.40; $P = .79$), and 10-year OS estimates were approximately 80% in both study arms. Regarding safety, RM was associated with a higher rate of grade 3 to 4 adverse events (24% vs 17%; $P = .0026$): cytopenias and infections were the only 2 adverse events observed with a higher frequency with the use of RM (4% vs 1% for both, respectively, in the RM and observation arms). QoL was similar in both study arms, suggesting bearable repeated rituximab infusions over 2 years for patients. In another study, RM after CVP but without rituximab as part of induction also improved PFS but not OS.[24]

RITUXIMAB MAINTENANCE AFTER AUTOLOGOUS STEM CELL TRANSPLANT

RM after high-dose chemotherapy and autologous stem cell transplant (HDC-ASCT) was assessed in a phase III study conducted by the European Society for Blood and Marrow Transplantation (ClinicalTrials.gov number NCT00005589) in 280 rituximab-naive chemosensitive relapsed patients with FL.[25] After a median follow-up of 8.3 years, RM after HDC-ASCT showed a significant improvement in 10-year PFS compared with observation (54% vs 37%, respectively; $P = .012$) but not OS. Another single-center study suggested a benefit of RM after ASCT.[26]

META-ANALYSIS OF THE RANDOMIZED STUDIES

Vidal and colleagues[27] performed a meta-analysis of individual patient data from 11 randomized controlled trials comparing RM therapy with no maintenance (observation or RR) for patients with FL. Data for 2315 patients with FL were available for the meta-analysis of OS. In accordance with a previous summary-data–based meta-analysis,[28,29] patients receiving RM had an improved OS (pooled HR of death = 0.79; 95% CI, 0.66–0.96) compared with those who did not receive RM. The improvement in OS with RM was consistent across patients with different characteristics (age, performance status, Ann Arbor stage, FLIPI score, presence of a 7-cm bulk tumor) and having received rituximab as part of induction before RM. Similarly, patients who achieved either a CR or a PR also had significant OS improvement. However, when examining patient subgroups, patients receiving RM as second-line therapy showed a significant OS benefit, whereas those receiving RM as a consolidation of first-line therapy did not seem to have an OS benefit. The risk of adverse events was higher with RM, especially grade 3 to 4 infections (4.9% vs 7.1% in the observation and RM groups, respectively; HR = 1.27; 95% CI, 1.12–1.45). Overall, this meta-analysis underlines the potential benefit of RM for improving the OS of patients with FL, although it remains unproved whether this benefit also exists from the use of RM after R-chemo in first-line therapy. The weight of PRIMA data in this meta-analysis certainly accounts for this last finding.

REMAINING OPEN QUESTIONS
Optimal Schedule and Duration of Rituximab Maintenance

Various dosing schedules and treatment durations have been investigated over the years but never compared head to head. Although rituximab (375 mg/m^2) was administered every 2 months in the PRIMA, RWW (Rituximab versus Watch and Wait), and SAKK 35/08 studies,[12,14,22] the RESORT[18] and the EORTC intergroup[19] studies applied single infusions every 3 months. In the German Low-grade Lymphoma Study Group (GLSG)[21] and the Minnie Pearl Cancer Research Network[17] studies, rituximab was administered once a week for 4 consecutive weeks, given at 3 and 9 months or every 6 months for 2 years, respectively. Regarding pharmacokinetic data, a scheme consisting of a single infusion of rituximab at a dose of 375 mg/m^2/d every 2 months may be optimal to allow a residual, presumably more active, MoAb serum level between 2 infusions.[30–32] Likewise, the optimal duration for RM therapy currently remains unknown. In most studies, the duration of RM ranged from 6 months to 2 years, only the RESORT study[18] delivering RM until progression and the SAKK 35/03[15] for 5 years. However, the results of these trials and of the as-yet unpublished StiL (Study Group Indolent Lymphomas) NHL7-2008 MAINTAIN study suggest that side effects observed when RM is used for more than 2 years are more frequent and hence could counterbalance the benefit in delaying tumor progression (Rummel, unpublished data, 2019).

Toxicities

RM therapy has been shown to be associated with grade 3 to 4 adverse events, mainly cytopenias and infections.[22,27] However, RM treatment is generally well tolerated, and these adverse events are easily manageable. RM leads to a transitional decrease in immunoglobulin G levels attributable to profound B-cell depletion. However, immunoglobulin substitution is not frequently used when first-line patients having received RM are considered. Although a very rare event, a few cases of fatal PML were described during RM. Overall, it is worth noting that RM should be administered with caution in patients with FL, whose OS remains excellent. In cases of recurrent low-grade or emergent severe toxicity, especially infection, discontinuation of RM should be considered.

Subcutaneous Administration

Subcutaneous (SC) rituximab has been shown to be pharmacokinetically noninferior to intravenous (IV) administration if given at a fixed dose of 1400 mg SC.[33] Moreover, Davies and colleagues[34] showed similar safety and efficacy profiles of SC and IV rituximab when given as maintenance therapy. Thus, SC administration of rituximab is a valid and convenient option for patients receiving maintenance therapy.

Rituximab Maintenance After Bendamustine-Based Induction Treatment

In recent years, bendamustine has become one of the favorite cytotoxic agents for use in combination with rituximab in the first-line treatment of patients with FL.[35,36] However, the effect of RM after bendamustine-rituximab (B-R) induction treatment has never been evaluated in randomized studies. The results of the GALLIUM study showed a higher and unexpected incidence of fatal toxicities in patients receiving anti-CD20 (either rituximab or obinutuzumab) maintenance therapy after bendamustine-containing induction.[37,38] It is also known that bendamustine induces a depletion of T lymphocytes that may expose patients to additional toxicities and compromise some of the anti-CD20 immune-mediated antitumor effects. However, indirect evidence coming from both the BRIGHT study[39] and a recent retrospective analysis[40] indicates that RM may provide a PFS benefit in patients who received B-R as induction therapy. The BRIGHT report suggested that this clinical benefit might only apply to patients in PR after B-R.

Cost-Effectiveness

The question of RM cost-effectiveness seems to be an important clinical parameter to determine the beneficial impact of such a treatment schedule given the absence of clear OS benefit. In 2012, Hornberger and colleagues[41] assessed the cost-effectiveness of RM compared with observation estimating PFS and OS over a representative patient's lifetime. Analysis was performed from the reported outcome of the PRIMA study. The incremental cost-effectiveness ratio per quality-adjusted life year was within the range of acceptable cost-effectiveness in the United States. The authorized use of rituximab biosimilars will undoubtedly improve the cost-effectiveness of maintenance treatment.

Using a Response-to-Treatment Individualized Approach to Administer Rituximab Maintenance

Despite the fact that RM seemed equally effective in helping patients achieving a CR or a PR after induction therapy in several studies, new response criteria such as PET/computed tomography (CT) or molecular minimal residual disease (MRD) evaluation might help to identify a group of patients who may have a deeper response after induction and for whom RM may not add a PFS benefit. In particular, patients who have achieved a PET-CT metabolic response seem in several studies to have an excellent outcome.[42,43] Recently, the Italian FOLL12 trial compared standard RM versus response-adapted RM in newly diagnosed patients with FL requiring first-line immunochemotherapy treatment.[44] An interim analysis revealed a significantly inferior estimated 3-year PFS in the response-adapted experimental arm (patients with CR by PET-CT and/or MRD results), thus leading to stoppage of the study. These data support the favorable effect on PFS of RM after induction therapy regardless of the depth of metabolic response assessed by PET-CT after induction. Another study (PETReA, Eudract 2016-004010-10) currently in recruitment has a similar design.

SUMMARY

Because patients with FL usually experience disease recurrence after each treatment line, offering maintenance treatment seems to be an attractive option to prolong remission after an induction therapy. The ideal maintenance strategy would involve significant benefit, good tolerance, minimal side effects, and convenient administration. The safety of RM, the management of side effects, and the optimization of rituximab delivery using SC administration all constitute supportive arguments in favor of

RM. A limited duration and appropriate scheduling would probably also optimize the cost/benefit ratio of RM.

The relevant questions are related to (1) the potential effect of RM on the natural course of the disease and (2) whether it is worth prolonging a treatment in patients with FL without improving OS. In the PRIMA study, the rate of progression with disease transformation was low in both arms, and RM did not delay the time to transformation.[22,23] However, in a compilation of multiple patient series, both rituximab induction and maintenance seemed to significantly reduce the rate of histologic transformation.[45] The 10-year cumulative hazard of histologic transformation was 5.9% for patients who received RI only and 3.6% (95% CI, 2.3–5.5) for those treated with induction and RM, suggesting that the use of RM may reduce the risk of transformation (HR, 0.55; 95% CI, 0.37–0.81; $P = .003$).

Despite highly significant improvements in PFS (or EFS) in patients with various characteristics and at various lines of therapy, only a few individual maintenance trials have suggested a trend toward improved survival for the RM arm, and none of them showed an unequivocal OS benefit in the long-term follow-up. However, the meta-analysis based on individual patient data clearly showed an improvement of OS with RM regardless of patient and disease characteristics and regardless of the induction treatment.[27] A direct extrapolation of PFS as a surrogate marker for OS cannot be made in FL even with long-term follow-up, which is likely related to the indolent nature of the disease but also to the efficacy of a variety of second-line or salvage treatments, resulting altogether in a prolonged survival expectancy of patients with current treatment standards.

Overall, the choice to apply RM in the context of the wide treatment landscape available for patients with FL should be guided by the evidence-based data reported earlier but should also result from an unbiased physician-patient discussion. Although the lack of clear OS benefit for patients treated in the first-line setting provides an argument against RM, the long treatment-free intervals observed in studies such as SAKK 35/98 and PRIMA offer patients the hope to live without symptoms for years despite the (still limited) burden associated with this treatment.

DISCLOSURE

G. Salles has received honoraria for participation in educational events or advisory boards from Roche/Genentech.

REFERENCES

1. Swenson WT, Wooldridge JE, Lynch CF, et al. Improved survival of follicular lymphoma patients in the United States. J Clin Oncol 2005;23(22):5019–26.

2. Casulo C, Nastoupil L, Fowler NH, et al. Unmet needs in the first-line treatment of follicular lymphoma. Ann Oncol 2017;28(9):2094–106.

3. Ezdinli EZ, Harrington DP, Kucuk O, et al. The effect of intensive intermittent maintenance therapy in advanced low-grade non-Hodgkin's lymphoma. Cancer 1987; 60(2):156–60.

4. Steward WP, Crowther D, McWilliam LJ, et al. Maintenance chlorambucil after CVP in the management of advanced stage, low-grade histologic type non-Hodgkin's lymphoma. A randomized prospective study with an assessment of prognostic factors. Cancer 1988;61(3):441–7.

5. Rohatiner AZS, Gregory WM, Peterson B, et al. Meta-analysis to evaluate the role of interferon in follicular lymphoma. J Clin Oncol 2005;23(10):2215–23.

6. Cartron G, Watier H, Golay J, et al. From the bench to the bedside: ways to improve rituximab efficacy. Blood 2004;104(9):2635–42.
7. Selenko N, Majdic O, Jäger U, et al. Cross-priming of cytotoxic T cells promoted by apoptosis-inducing tumor cell reactive antibodies? J Clin Immunol 2002;22(3): 124–30.
8. Hilchey SP, Hyrien O, Mosmann TR, et al. Rituximab immunotherapy results in the induction of a lymphoma idiotype-specific T-cell response in patients with follicular lymphoma: support for a "vaccinal effect" of rituximab. Blood 2009; 113(16):3809–12.
9. Roulland S, Navarro J-M, Grenot P, et al. Follicular lymphoma-like B cells in healthy individuals: a novel intermediate step in early lymphomagenesis. J Exp Med 2006;203(11):2425–31.
10. Hainsworth JD, Litchy S, Burris HA, et al. Rituximab as first-line and maintenance therapy for patients with indolent non-hodgkin's lymphoma. J Clin Oncol 2002; 20(20):4261–7.
11. McLaughlin P, Grillo-López AJ, Link BK, et al. Rituximab chimeric anti-CD20 monoclonal antibody therapy for relapsed indolent lymphoma: half of patients respond to a four-dose treatment program. J Clin Oncol 1998;16(8):2825–33.
12. Ghielmini M, Schmitz S-FH, Cogliatti SB, et al. Prolonged treatment with rituximab in patients with follicular lymphoma significantly increases event-free survival and response duration compared with the standard weekly x 4 schedule. Blood 2004; 103(12):4416–23.
13. Martinelli G, Schmitz S-FH, Utiger U, et al. Long-term follow-up of patients with follicular lymphoma receiving single-agent rituximab at two different schedules in trial SAKK 35/98. J Clin Oncol 2010;28(29):4480–4.
14. Ardeshna KM, Qian W, Smith P, et al. Rituximab versus a watch-and-wait approach in patients with advanced-stage, asymptomatic, non-bulky follicular lymphoma: an open-label randomised phase 3 trial. Lancet Oncol 2014;15(4): 424–35.
15. Taverna C, Martinelli G, Hitz F, et al. Rituximab maintenance for a maximum of 5 years after single-agent rituximab induction in follicular lymphoma: results of the randomized controlled phase III Trial SAKK 35/03. J Clin Oncol 2016;34(5): 495–500.
16. Davis TA, Grillo-López AJ, White CA, et al. Rituximab anti-CD20 monoclonal antibody therapy in non-Hodgkin's lymphoma: safety and efficacy of re-treatment. J Clin Oncol 2000;18(17):3135–43.
17. Hainsworth JD, Litchy S, Shaffer DW, et al. Maximizing therapeutic benefit of rituximab: maintenance therapy versus re-treatment at progression in patients with indolent non-Hodgkin's lymphoma–a randomized phase II trial of the Minnie Pearl Cancer Research Network. J Clin Oncol 2005;23(6):1088–95.
18. Kahl BS, Hong F, Williams ME, et al. Rituximab extended schedule or re-treatment trial for low-tumor burden follicular lymphoma: eastern cooperative oncology group protocol e4402. J Clin Oncol 2014;32(28):3096–102.
19. van Oers MHJ, Klasa R, Marcus RE, et al. Rituximab maintenance improves clinical outcome of relapsed/resistant follicular non-Hodgkin lymphoma in patients both with and without rituximab during induction: results of a prospective randomized phase 3 intergroup trial. Blood 2006;108(10):3295–301.
20. van Oers MHJ, Van Glabbeke M, Giurgea L, et al. Rituximab maintenance treatment of relapsed/resistant follicular non-Hodgkin's lymphoma: long-term outcome of the EORTC 20981 phase III randomized intergroup study. J Clin Oncol 2010; 28(17):2853–8.

21. Forstpointner R, Unterhalt M, Dreyling M, et al. Maintenance therapy with rituximab leads to a significant prolongation of response duration after salvage therapy with a combination of rituximab, fludarabine, cyclophosphamide, and mitoxantrone (R-FCM) in patients with recurring and refractory follicular and mantle cell lymphomas: results of a prospective randomized study of the German Low Grade Lymphoma Study Group (GLSG). Blood 2006;108(13):4003–8.

22. Salles G, Seymour JF, Offner F, et al. Rituximab maintenance for 2 years in patients with high tumour burden follicular lymphoma responding to rituximab plus chemotherapy (PRIMA): a phase 3, randomised controlled trial. Lancet 2011;377(9759):42–51.

23. Bachy E, Seymour JF, Feugier P, et al. Sustained progression-free survival benefit of rituximab maintenance in patients with follicular lymphoma: long-term results of the PRIMA study. J Clin Oncol 2019;JCO1901073. https://doi.org/10.1200/JCO.19.01073.

24. Barta SK, Li H, Hochster HS, et al. Randomized phase 3 study in low-grade lymphoma comparing maintenance anti-CD20 antibody with observation after induction therapy: a trial of the ECOG-ACRIN Cancer Research Group (E1496). Cancer 2016;122(19):2996–3004.

25. Pettengell R, Schmitz N, Gisselbrecht C, et al. Rituximab purging and/or maintenance in patients undergoing autologous transplantation for relapsed follicular lymphoma: a prospective randomized trial from the lymphoma working party of the European group for blood and marrow transplantation. J Clin Oncol 2013;31(13):1624–30.

26. Bourcier J, Gastinne T, Leux C, et al. Rituximab maintenance after autologous stem cell transplantation prolongs response duration in non-naive rituximab follicular lymphoma patients: a single institution experience. Ann Hematol 2016;95(8):1287–93.

27. Vidal L, Gafter-Gvili A, Salles G, et al. Rituximab maintenance improves overall survival of patients with follicular lymphoma-Individual patient data meta-analysis. Eur J Cancer 2017;76:216–25.

28. Vidal L, Gafter-Gvili A, Leibovici L, et al. Rituximab maintenance for the treatment of patients with follicular lymphoma: systematic review and meta-analysis of randomized trials. J Natl Cancer Inst 2009;101(4):248–55.

29. Vidal L, Gafter-Gvili A, Salles G, et al. Rituximab maintenance for the treatment of patients with follicular lymphoma: an updated systematic review and meta-analysis of randomized trials. J Natl Cancer Inst 2011;103(23):1799–806.

30. Berinstein NL, Grillo-López AJ, White CA, et al. Association of serum Rituximab (IDEC-C2B8) concentration and anti-tumor response in the treatment of recurrent low-grade or follicular non-Hodgkin's lymphoma. Ann Oncol 1998;9(9):995–1001.

31. Gordan LN, Grow WB, Pusateri A, et al. Phase II trial of individualized rituximab dosing for patients with CD20-positive lymphoproliferative disorders. J Clin Oncol 2005;23(6):1096–102.

32. Jäger U, Fridrik M, Zeitlinger M, et al. Rituximab serum concentrations during immuno-chemotherapy of follicular lymphoma correlate with patient gender, bone marrow infiltration and clinical response. Haematologica 2012;97(9):1431–8.

33. Salar A, Avivi I, Bittner B, et al. Comparison of subcutaneous versus intravenous administration of rituximab as maintenance treatment for follicular lymphoma: results from a two-stage, phase IB study. J Clin Oncol 2014;32(17):1782–91.

34. Davies A, Merli F, Mihaljević B, et al. Efficacy and safety of subcutaneous rituximab versus intravenous rituximab for first-line treatment of follicular lymphoma

(SABRINA): a randomised, open-label, phase 3 trial. Lancet Haematol 2017;4(6): e272–82.

35. Rummel MJ, Niederle N, Maschmeyer G, et al. Bendamustine plus rituximab versus CHOP plus rituximab as first-line treatment for patients with indolent and mantle-cell lymphomas: an open-label, multicentre, randomised, phase 3 non-inferiority trial. Lancet 2013;381(9873):1203–10.

36. Flinn IW, van der Jagt R, Kahl B, et al. First-line treatment of patients with indolent non-hodgkin lymphoma or mantle-cell lymphoma with bendamustine plus rituximab versus R-CHOP or R-CVP: results of the BRIGHT 5-year follow-up study. J Clin Oncol 2019;37(12):984–91.

37. Marcus R, Seymour JF, Hiddemann W. Obinutuzumab treatment of follicular lymphoma. N Engl J Med 2017;377(26):2605–6.

38. Hiddemann W, Barbui AM, Canales MA, et al. Immunochemotherapy with obinutuzumab or rituximab for previously untreated follicular lymphoma in the GALLIUM study: influence of chemotherapy on efficacy and safety. J Clin Oncol 2018;36(23):2395–404.

39. Kahl BS, Burke JM, van der Jagt R, et al. Assessment of maintenance rituximab after first-line bendamustine-rituximab in patients with follicular lymphoma: an analysis from the BRIGHT trial. Blood 2017;130(Supplement 1):484.

40. Hill BT, Nastoupil L, Winter AM, et al. Maintenance rituximab or observation after frontline treatment with bendamustine-rituximab for follicular lymphoma. Br J Haematol 2019;184(4):524–35.

41. Hornberger J, Chien R, Friedmann M, et al. Cost-effectiveness of rituximab as maintenance therapy in patients with follicular non-Hodgkin lymphoma after responding to first-line rituximab plus chemotherapy. Leuk Lymphoma 2012; 53(12):2371–7.

42. Trotman J, Fournier M, Lamy T, et al. Positron emission tomography-computed tomography (PET-CT) after induction therapy is highly predictive of patient outcome in follicular lymphoma: analysis of PET-CT in a subset of PRIMA trial participants. J Clin Oncol 2011;29(23):3194–200.

43. Trotman J, Barrington SF, Belada D, et al. Prognostic value of end-of-induction PET response after first-line immunochemotherapy for follicular lymphoma (GALLIUM): secondary analysis of a randomised, phase 3 trial. Lancet Oncol 2018;19(11):1530–42.

44. Federico M. Response oriented maintenance therapy in advanced follicular lymphoma. Results of the interim analysis of the FOLL12 trial conducted by Fondazione italiana Linfomi. Hematol Oncol 2019;37(S2):153–4.

45. Federico M, Caballero Barrigón MD, Marcheselli L, et al. Rituximab and the risk of transformation of follicular lymphoma: a retrospective pooled analysis. Lancet Haematol 2018;5(8):e359–67.

Cellular Therapy in Follicular Lymphoma

Autologous Stem Cell Transplantation, Allogeneic Stem Cell Transplantation, and Chimeric Antigen Receptor T-cell Therapy

Jessica Okosun, MB, BChir, PhD[a], Silvia Montoto, MD[b],*

KEYWORDS

- Follicular lymphoma • Stem cell transplantation • Adoptive therapy • CAR T cell

KEY POINTS

- Autologous stem cell transplantation (ASCT) is an efficacious treatment option for patients with relapsed follicular lymphoma (FL), especially those with early progression, which is capable of inducing long-term remissions.
- Although potentially curative, allogeneic transplantation has not shown superiority to ASCT and should be reserved for selected patients with relapse post-ASCT or those with high-risk FL.
- Emerging early-phase data point to promising response rates with chimeric antigen receptor T-cell therapy.
- With numerous competing nontransplant options, robust clinical and biological features that identify patients who will most benefit from these therapies remain an area of unmet need.

INTRODUCTION

Outcomes for follicular lymphoma (FL) have continued to improve with each decade. A subset of high-risk FL patients, however, in particular those who have early relapse, are refractory to conventional therapies, and those with high-grade transformation continue to pose a therapeutic dilemma, with limited treatment options and lack of established consensus strategies. Cellular, or cell, therapy refers to the transfer of

[a] Centre for Haemato-Oncology, Barts Cancer Institute, Queen Mary University of London, John Vane Science Centre, Charterhouse Square, London EC1M 6BQ, UK; [b] Department of Haemato-Oncology, St Bartholomew's Hospital, London, UK
* Corresponding author. Department of Haemato-Oncology, St Bartholomew's Hospital, West Smithfield, London EC1A 7BE, UK.
E-mail address: s.montoto@qmul.ac.uk

Hematol Oncol Clin N Am 34 (2020) 701–714
https://doi.org/10.1016/j.hoc.2020.02.006
0889-8588/20/© 2020 Elsevier Inc. All rights reserved.

live cells that may have been selected, expanded, or modified ex vivo before administration into a patient to provide therapeutic benefit. The most frequently used cellular therapy, hematopoietic stem cell (HSC) transplantation, has been around since the 1960s and, in the context of lymphomas, represented an alternative option for those that had failed conventional therapies, offering potential curative options either through high-dose therapy supported by autologous stem cell transplantation (ASCT) or allogeneic stem cell transplantation (alloSCT). Over the past decade, an exciting phase has been encountered, with the next generation of emergent adoptive cell therapies, where autologous T cells are manipulated ex vivo and reinfused back into the patient to generate an immune-mediated antitumor response, such as chimeric antigen receptor (CAR) T-cell therapy and tumor-infiltrating lymphocytes (TILs). This review discusses the up-to-date data on stem cell transplantation (SCT), both autologous and allogeneic, as well as emergent CAR T-cell therapies and where they potentially fit into the treatment armamentarium for patients with FL.

AUTOLOGOUS STEM CELL TRANSPLANTATION IN FOLLICULAR LYMPHOMA
Is There a Role for Consolidation in First Remission?

The merit of upfront high-dose therapy with ASCT as a consolidation of first remission is limited, because no improvements in overall survival (OS) were reported in any of the randomized studies conducted during the prerituximab era[1–4] or in the only study undertaken in the postrituximab era.[5] Although there was demonstrated benefit in progression-free survival (PFS) in 3 of the studies, there were significant toxicities and, in particular, an increase in secondary malignancies (such as myelodysplastic syndrome [MDS] and acute myeloid leukemia [AML]) in the ASCT arm.[1,2,5] In addition, as discussed previously, no evidence was detected on OS in any of the trials, because many of the patients randomized to the nontransplant arm did receive ASCT at a later relapse, neutralizing the potential benefit of ASCT in first remission. On the basis of these data, routine use of ASCT as consolidation after first remission cannot be recommended.

Autologous Stem Cell Transplantation for Relapsed/Refractory Follicular Lymphoma

By contrast, there has been a single prospective randomized study in the relapsed setting that compared conventional chemotherapy alone (C) versus chemotherapy followed by ASCT using either unpurged (U) or purged (P) stem cell harvests in relapsed FL patients (CUP trial). Although the trial closed prematurely due to poor accrual, it demonstrated a significant benefit in clinical outcomes. The 2-year PFS rates were 26%, 58%, and 55% for the C, U, and P arms, respectively, together with a correspondingly positive impact on OS for the transplant arms, with 4-year OS rates of 46%, 71%, and 77%, respectively.[6] The direct clinical relevance of this study in the modern era remains debatable, because it was conducted prior to the advent of the current chemoimmunotherapy approaches. Additionally, there have been several non-randomized retrospective studies utilizing ASCT spanning the prerituximab to rituximab eras that have shown efficacy for the long-term control of FL.[7–10] The challenges in the collective interpretation of these studies have been the wide variability in several factors that can have an impact on response: selection of patient cohorts (rituximab-naïve vs rituximab-experienced and the time point of rituximab use: as initial treatment or at relapse, as part of induction or as maintenance), the type of salvage and conditioning regimes used, and the pretransplant remission status. Although it is impossible to normalize these variations across the studies, it appears that 5-year PFS is approximately 50% to 60% and 5-year OS greater than 50%. With the exception of rituximab-refractory patients, there is benefit of rituximab usage during salvage treatment because this demonstrates improved outcome post-ASCT.[9,11] Recent studies with long-term follow-up data have reported a plateau in PFS after ASCT, with 10-year PFS of approximately 30% to 35%, suggesting that this approach not only was effective in producing durable remissions but also is potentially curative for a subset of relapsed FL patients.[12–14] Receiving maintenance rituximab further augments this observation with the most recent update of the phase III European Society for Blood and Marrow Transplantation (EBMT) LYM1 trial reporting a superior 10-year PFS of 58% in patients who received maintenance rituximab post-ASCT compared with those who did not.[15]

At present, there is no universal recommendation on the indications and optimal timing of ASCT during a patient's disease course. The consensus project of the EBMT-Lymphoma Working Party (LWP-EBMT), however, recommends ASCT as a consolidation strategy in patients with a first chemosensitive FL relapse, especially with high-risk features, such as high-risk FLIPI score or short duration of response after chemoimmunotherapy[16] or as an option in those with second or subsequent relapses.[17,18]

Autologous Stem Cell Transplantation for Early Relapsed and Transformed Follicular Lymphoma

Although considered incurable, the outcomes for FL patients have continually improved, with median survival now approaching 2 decades.[19] There are subsets of patients with high-risk disease characterized by a significantly poorer survival. These include patients with early relapse within the first 2 years after induction chemoimmunotherapy (referred to as progression of disease at 24 months) and those with transformed disease after prior treatment of nontransformed FL, altogether believed to represent approximately 15% to 20% of the FL population.[20,21] The data imply a clear role for ASCT for those with early progression or chemorefractoriness. A retrospective subset analysis of ASCT in 655 patients with relapsed FL from the GELTAMO (Spanish Lymphoma and Bone Marrow Transplant Group) study group registry reported that 87 patients with progression of disease at 24 months who underwent ASCT in either second complete response or second partial response had 5-year PFS and OS rates of 43% and 69%, respectively.[22] This cohort consisted of patients that were all rituximab-naïve, not representative of the majority of early progressed FL patients seen with current practices. Similarly, the German Low Grade Lymphoma Study Group confirmed that ASCT in early relapsed rituximab-naïve FL patients resulted in significantly higher 5-year OS compared with those not receiving ASCT (77% vs 46%, respectively).[23] A joint National LymphoCare Study and the Center for International Blood and Marrow Transplant Research (CIBMTR) retrospective study evaluated patients experiencing early therapy failure who received prior frontline rituximab-based chemoimmunotherapy comparing 2 patient cohorts, 1 receiving ASCT (n = 175 patients) and the other receiving non-ASCT treatment (n = 174). There was no difference in 5-year OS between the 2 cohorts (60% vs 67%, respectively; $P = .16$); however, the early use of ASCT less than 1 year after treatment failure was associated with a higher 5-year OS compared with those without an ASCT (73% vs 60%, respectively; $P = .05$), advocating the benefit of early consolidation with ASCT.[24]

For transformed FL (tFL), retrospective series indicate that consolidative ASCT is beneficial. A multicenter Danish study reported superior PFS and OS for patients receiving ASCT compared with those receiving rituximab-chemotherapy alone (5-year PFS 53% vs 6%, respectively; 5-year OS 62% vs 36%, respectively).[25] After a median follow-up of 6 years, 40 patients from the PRIMA (Primary Rituximab and Maintenance) trial had histologic transformation after immunochemotherapy and rituximab maintenance, with those receiving ASCT presenting an improved OS compared with those without (median performance status, not reached vs 1.7 years).[26] Given the infrequent nature of tFL, particularly in the rituximab era, there have been no randomized or prospective studies addressing this question. Nevertheless, it is viewed that autologous transplantation remains an appropriate option for those with prior treatment of their un-transformed FL.[27]

ALLOGENEIC STEM CELL TRANSPLANTATION

Myeloablative alloSCT offers the possibility of a cure for FL, with compelling evidence for a strong graft versus lymphoma effect. It incurs considerable morbidity and mortality risks, however, which outweigh the potential beneficial effect of a myeloablative alloSCT. Hence, this is rarely indicated in patients with FL. Given the median age of FL patients, nonmyeloablative (reduced intensity conditioning [RIC]) approaches increasingly have been utilized for relapsed FL, with a significant reduction in the nonrelapse mortality (NRM).[28–33] These studies, however, have reported diverse outcomes due to the inherent heterogeneity of the cohorts in terms of reporting on differing patient populations and treatment characteristics. Allowing for differences in study populations, most of the published reports quote a 3-year transplant-related mortality rate of 20% to 30%, with a 3-year PFS rate of 50% to 60% and a 3-year OS rate of 50% to 65%. The MD Anderson Cancer Center series published by Khouri and colleagues[29] reported significantly better results in the setting of a prospective phase II trial, with estimated OS and PFS of 85% and 83%, respectively, after a median follow-up of 60 months. In this study, a majority of the patients received a transplant from a matched sibling donor (45 of 47) and only 19% had relapsed after a previous ASCT, which could, at least partially, contribute to these excellent results. There have been attempts to identify population groups who clearly would benefit from alloSCT. Not surprisingly, age, performance status, number of prior lines of therapy, and chemosensitivity all are factors that have an impact on the outcome after alloSCT,[34] but there is not a distinctive subgroup of patients with relapsed FL in whom alloSCT seems to be the strategy of choice. International recommendations support the use of alloSCT in patients relapsing after an ASCT.[16] Surprisingly, there are not many articles focusing on the role of alloSCT in patients who relapsed after an ASCT. The LWP-EBMT reported on 183 patients who received RIC-alloSCT for FL relapsed post-ASCT. After median follow-up of approximately 5 years, 2-year NRM was 27%, with 5-year PFS and OS of approximately 50%. For most of the patients, the response duration after alloSCT was longer than the previous response duration after ASCT.[35]

Autologous Stem Cell Transplantation Versus Allogeneic Stem Cell Transplantation

One of the main questions regarding the role of SCT in the management of patients with FL is, What should the modality of choice be for a first SCT, ASCT or alloSCT? The curative potential of alloSCT is counteracted by a still high rate of NRM, even with RIC-alloSCT, whereas ASCT is a much safer procedure but associated with a higher relapse rate. Several retrospective (mostly registry) studies have tried to answer this question, but the different characteristics of the patients in the 2 cohorts, in terms of previous lines of therapy and response to treatment (which are prognostic factors), make it difficult to draw firm conclusions. The LWP-EBMT compared the outcomes of 726 patients with FL who had an ASCT with that of 149 patients who had RIC-alloSCT as the first SCT.[36] Not surprisingly, alloSCT was associated with a significantly higher

NRM, whereas ASCT resulted in a higher relapse rate. This resulted in a lack of significant differences in OS or PFS (although, after 2 years of follow-up, patients in the RIC-alloSCT group seem to benefit from a PFS advantage). A prospective clinical trial attempted to answer this question in a randomized fashion (ClinicalTrials.gov number, NCT00096460). The Blood and Marrow Transplant Clinical Trials Network conducted a multicenter trial in patients with relapsed FL with a biological assignment to ASCT or alloSCT depending on donor availability.[37] Unfortunately, the trial was closed less than 2 years after its opening due to slow enrollment, having recruited only 30 patients. For high-risk FL, a retrospective CIBMTR analyses on 141 biopsy-proved tFL, who underwent SCT, demonstrated a significantly higher NRM in those who received alloSCT compared with ASCT (1-year NRM: 41% vs 8%, respectively) neutralizing any benefit from alloSCT (5-year OS: 22% for alloSCT and 50% for ASCT).[38] Similarly, an analyses of more than 400 patients with early relapse within 24 months of chemoimmunotherapy showed no difference in OS between ASCT and matched sibling alloSCT (5-year OS: 70% vs 73%, respectively) with a significantly lower 5-year NRM of 5% for ASCT and 17% for matched sibling alloSCT.[39]

Long-Term Sequelae of Hematopoietic Stem Cell Transplantation—New Considerations

Although ASCT provides durable remissions for patients with relapsed FL, it is important to recognize the accompanying risk of long-term toxicities. A major concern is the late risk of developing secondary malignancies, in particular myeloid malignancies, MDS and AML, which have been a common cause of NRM. This increased risk occurs particularly when total body irradiation conditioning was used, an approach that now is rarely adopted.[40,41] Retrospective analyses of FL patients who underwent ASCT in the Spanish GELTAMO registry reported 12.75% of patients developing secondary malignancies, thus translating to a 3.1-fold higher risk of developing secondary malignancy compared with the general population. Notably, 40% of these malignancies were AML or MDS, with the survival after these diagnoses considerably shortened to a median of only 1.25 years.[42]

Critically, in the past 5 years, there has been increasing evidence showing that with age, 1 or more somatic mutations are accumulated in the hematopoietic stem cells (HSCs) that confer a competitive advantage. The clonal progeny of these mutant HSCs thus are detected in the peripheral blood, a condition referred to as clonal hematopoiesis (CH) or age-related clonal hematopoiesis.[43,44] The presence of CH is associated with a higher propensity to develop myeloid neoplasms and cardiovascular disease.[44,45] Approximately 20% to 30% of people older than 60 years of age have CH.[46,47] Given the median age of patients with FL at diagnosis, it may be expected that a proportion of patients could harbor a clonal HSC population with CH-associated mutations at the time of stem cell apheresis. It appears that the presence of CH can have a negative impact on outcomes after ASCT. In 30% of patients with non-Hodgkin lymphoma (NHL) who underwent ASCT, Gibson and colleagues[48] identified CH mutations at the time of their transplant, in particular mutations in *TP53* and *PPM1D*. Having CH mutations at the time of the ASCT was associated with a greater than 3-fold increased risk of therapy-related myeloid neoplasms (14.1% for those with CH vs 4.3% those without CH) and this correlated with a significantly inferior OS (10-y OS 30.4% vs 60.9%, respectively). A study demonstrated that 6.3% of stem cell harvests from donors greater than 55 years of age for alloSCT in recipients with lymphoid malignancies harbored CH mutations. The presence of donor graft CH mutations did not result in inferior recipient survival rates, albeit with a higher incidence of graft-versus-host disease; however the numbers of lymphoma-associated transplants in this study were small.[49] Recent studies suggest that cytotoxic therapy and ASCT act as hematopoietic stressors that subsequently promote the selective engraftment and expansion of these preexisting mutant CH clones.[50,51] Prospective studies are warranted to validate these observations and determine the relevance of CH mutations in this context. Nevertheless, these findings raise the question on whether integrating analyses for CH mutations into pre-HSC transplantation screening and risk prediction assessments is needed to optimally prevent or manage late complications associated with HSC transplantation.

ADOPTIVE CELLULAR THERAPY: CHIMERIC ANTIGEN RECEPTOR T CELLS

The basic structure of CARs comprises an extracellular antigen-recognition domain (usually a single-chain variable fragment generated from a monoclonal antibody targeting a specific tumor associated antigen) that is anchored to the cell via a transmembrane hinge. This extracellular domain is fused via the hinge to an intracellular domain that usually is the CD3 zeta chain of the T-cell receptor, which is critical for TCR signaling. The extracellular domain of the CAR permits the recognition of a specific antigen by T cells and the signaling domain subsequently stimulates T-cell proliferation, cytokine secretion, and ultimately T-cell activation. First-generation CARs typically utilized the CD3 signaling chain to provide the activation signal; however, these demonstrated limited efficacy in clinical trials, likely due to lack of long-term T-cell expansion. Second-generation CARs use the first-generation backbone but have increased potency because they contain a second costimulatory signaling molecule, such as CD28, 4-1BB, and OX-40. Therefore, upon encountering the tumor antigen, these second-generation CAR T cells deliver both activation (signal 1) and costimulatory signals (signal 2) to improve T-cell activation and antitumor potency. Although numerous tumor antigen targets are under investigation, the most advanced CAR T cells target the CD19 antigen that is expressed on the majority of B-cell malignancies, including B-NHL and B-cell acute lymphoblastic leukemia.

Efficacy of Chimeric Antigen Receptor T-cell Therapy in Follicular Lymphoma

No clinical efficacy in patients with FL cases was demonstrated with the first generation of anti-CD19 CAR T cells without costimulation.[52] Subsequently, second-generation anti-CD19 CAR T cells with CD28 costimulation resulted in a long-term remission in a refractory FL patient.[53] A phase II trial evaluating anti-CD19 CAR T cells with a 4-1BB costimulatory domain (CTL019, now known as tisagenlecleucel) in relapsed/refractory CD19$^+$ lymphomas (ClinicalTrials.gov number, NCT02030834) included 14 FL patients with progression of lymphoma less than 2 years after second or higher line of therapy. At 6 months, 10 of 14 patients (71%) were in complete remission (CR) and, at a median follow-up of 29 months, 70% were progression-free.[54] In the phase II JULIET trial evaluating tisagenlecleucel in relapsed/refractory diffuse large B-cell lymphoma (DLBCL), 21 of the 111 patients treated had tFL. A breakdown for outcomes based on histology was not performed. Here, the best overall response rate was 52%, with 40% CRs and, at 12 months after the initial response, the rate of relapse-free survival was 65%.[55] ZUMA-1, a phase II multicenter trial for axicabtagene ciloleucel, enrolled 111 patients with histologically confirmed DLBCL with refractory disease or progression/relapse within 12 months of an ASCT (101 received axicabtagene ciloleucel). In a cohort that included 16 patients with tFL and 8 with PMBCL, the overall response rate was 83% with CR seen in 71% of patients.[56]

More recently, Hirayama and colleagues[57] reported impressive response rates in an early-phase trial of 21 patients with relapsed/refractory FL (n = 8) and tFL (n = 13).

Approximately 50% of the cohort had been treated with a previous ASCT and 3 of the 21 patients had a previous alloSCT. Patients received cyclophosphamide and fludarabine lymphodepletion followed by infusion of 2×10^6 CD19 CAR T cells/kg, using the 4-1BB costimulatory domain as in tisagenlecleucel, but included a 1:1 ratio of $CD4^+$ to $CD8^+$ T cells. CR rates by the Lugano criteria were 88% and 46% for patients with FL and tFL, respectively. Durable remissions were demonstrated because all patients with FL who achieved CR remained in remission at a median follow-up of 24 months.[57]

Overall, these studies highlight promising activity, particularly in relapsed/refractory FL. Response rates for tFL appear similar to those in relapsed/refractory DLBCL, perhaps pointing to different biology between FL and tFL. Currently, anti-CD19 CAR T cell is an approved therapy for relapsed/refractory DLBCL, including tFL, in the United States. It is being actively evaluated in relapsed follicular and indolent NHL; for example, the phase II ZUMA-5 trial (ClinicalTrials.gov number, NCT03105336) aims to assess axicabtagene ciloleucel as treatment of indolent NHL that has relapsed or is resistant to standard therapy.

Chimeric Antigen Receptor T-cell Toxicities

The 2 main categories of toxicities associated with CAR T-cell therapy are well described: cytokine release syndrome (CRS) and neurotoxicity (referred to as CAR T-cell–related encephalopathy syndrome), that can be accompanied by organ damage. CRS is an excessive inflammatory response caused by overactivation of immune effector cells that leads to significant release and elevation of inflammatory cytokines, such as interleukin (IL)-2, IL-6, interferon-γ, and tumor necrosis factor, with typical symptoms experienced pyrexia, malaise, hypotension, and hypoxia, in a sense somewhat mimicking a systemic inflammatory response syndrome. In severe cases, irreversible end-organ dysfunction and death can occur. Products with CD28 costimulatory domains typically are associated with a greater incidence of severe neurotoxicity related to CRS, whereas the opposite is true for those using 4-1BB,[54,56] although the biological rationale for this is unclear. An anti–IL-6 receptor antibody, tocilizumab, together with corticosteroids, frequently is used to minimize the effects of CRS in patients. An anti–IL-6 monoclonal antibody, siltuximab, also can reduce the associated CRS. There is no evidence that either of these 2 treatments is superior and, importantly, they do not seem to affect the efficacy of CAR T-cell therapy.

Patients with neurotoxicity experience a range of symptoms, including confusion, headaches, tremor, and agitation. Some of the symptoms of neurotoxicity overlap with CRS. Similar to CRS, neurotoxicity appears to be cytokine-driven. Specific clinical factors appear to correlate with the development of CRS and neurotoxicity, such as disease burden, dose of CAR T cells administered, and cytokine profiles. There are ongoing efforts to understand the mechanisms and factors that contribute to these life-threatening toxicities in order to improve the safety of CAR T-cell therapy. For the most part, a majority of CAR T-cell–related toxicities resolve within a few weeks, although mortalities have also been reported. Early identification and grading of these potential complications are recommended. More recently, a defined criterion for measuring and grading CRS and neurotoxicity has been developed.[58,59]

OTHER EMERGING CELLULAR IMMUNOTHERAPIES

A proportion of patients fail to enter remission or relapse after receiving anti-CD19 CAR T-cell therapy. This has been attributed mostly to CAR T-cell resistance due to loss of the CD19 antigen and up-regulation of immune checkpoint molecules. Other modalities being developed to overcome anti-CD19 resistance and add to the CAR T-cell armamentarium include CAR T cells targeting alternate antigens like CD20,[60] dual CAR T cells that target 2 antigens to reduce the risk of developing antigen resistance,[61] and armoring CAR T cells that express immunomodulatory molecules to initiate endogenous immune response against the tumor thereby increasing its potency.[62] Beyond CAR T cells, experimental strategies with other adoptive cellular therapies are being tested. Ex vivo expansion and reinfusion of autologous TILs actually predate CAR T-cell therapy and have had clinical application and efficacy in select patients with metastatic melanoma.[63] Because the somatic mutations for most cancer types are now well defined, these mutations generate tumor-specific neoantigens that represent ideal targets for T-cell–based immunotherapies.[64] Neoantigen-directed therapies are being evaluated in clinical trials in a range of malignancies that utilize either TILs or cancer vaccines against specific neoantigens. A pilot study examining personalized cancer vaccines against individual tumor's neoantigens in FL patients who have only received rituximab is ongoing (ClinicalTrials.gov identifier: NCT03361852).

SEQUENCING CELLULAR THERAPIES AND FUTURE DIRECTIONS

There are challenges in sequencing therapies in FL, and these do not pertain only to cellular therapies. First, for a majority of patients, FL remains a disease that slowly progresses over a protracted clinical course. With a wealth of competing and rapidly emergent new therapies,[65] it has been difficult to develop a clear algorithm on how therapies should be sequenced. The cohorts that are best placed to benefit from cellular therapies have yet to be clearly defined. Data in CAR T-cell therapies in FL are still in their infancy, with long-term sequelae unknown; however, the early-phase data look promising. At present, most of the studies of ASCT, alloSCT, and CAR T-cell therapy typically are utilized in the setting of multiply relapsed or refractory FL or tFL. The current recommendations for these therapies are shown in **Table 1**. They maybe of greatest benefit earlier in the disease course or restricted purely to high-risk patients (early relapsed, chemorefractory, or tFL) but conducting large randomized trials is unlikely given the small subset of these patients. Currently, these decisions have to be weighed carefully on an individual patient basis, factoring in both immediate and long-term needs, risk factors, and toxicities of cellular therapy options against other existing noncellular therapies. Phase II trials in defined and selected patients could be appropriate, although the concern remains that cohorts who may benefit from transplantation strategies continue to reduce as these are supplanted by newer targeted therapies.

Detailed studies defining how best to identify patients at diagnoses or upon treatment initiation who will most benefit from cellular therapies or robust surrogate endpoints that reflect successful therapy currently are lacking. Although several predominantly clinical tools exist, such as FLIPI, FLIPI-2, and PRIMA-prognostic index, none as yet guides therapy,[66–68] and these tools cannot be implemented to capture every risk scenario. Tailored risk tools for specific scenarios are required. There has been an emphasis on defining risk upfront but tumor evolution driven inherently and/or with each therapy[69–71] means that dynamic risk assessment tools may be more appropriate to evaluate individual treatment strategy at each treatment-requiring juncture.

A good starting point may be to evaluate the precellular and postcellular therapy disease and biological characteristics of patients who attain long-term remissions to identify the features associated with the greatest benefit while in parallel examining

Table 1
Summary of indications and recommendations of cellular therapy options in follicular lymphoma

Cellular Therapy	Indications	Current Guidance	References
ASCT	Consolidation after first remission	Not recommended—EBMT	16–18
	For first relapse <2 y from diagnosis	Suitable consolidation option if stem cells available, low risk MDS/ AML	17,23,24
	For multiple relapses	Based on individual circumstances	16–18
AlloSCT	For first relapse <2 y from diagnosis	Not recommended if ASCT an available option Consider in highly selected younger patients with matched sibling donor available	18,38,39; NCCN guidelines for B-cell lymphomas, version 5, 2019
	For multiple relapses	For highly selected patients only	17,18
	Relapse post-ASCT	Should be considered	16,17
CAR T-cell	Failed ≥2 prior therapies	Axicabtagene ciloleucel or tisagenlecleucel, if not previously given for tFL only	NCCN guidelines for B-cell lymphomas version 5, 2019

Abbreviation: NCCN, National Comprehensive Cancer Network.

the features of those who fail such therapy early. Such a strategy may aid improved patient selection and personalized risk prediction and delineate the ultimate place and timing of cellular therapies in FL.

DISCLOSURE

The authors have nothing to disclose.

REFERENCES

1. Lenz G, Dreyling M, Schiegnitz E, et al. Myeloablative radiochemotherapy followed by autologous stem cell transplantation in first remission prolongs progression-free survival in follicular lymphoma: results of a prospective, randomized trial of the German Low-Grade Lymphoma Study Group. Blood 2004;104(9): 2667–74.

2. Deconinck E, Foussard C, Milpied N, et al. High-dose therapy followed by autologous purged stem-cell transplantation and doxorubicin-based chemotherapy in patients with advanced follicular lymphoma: a randomized multicenter study by GOELAMS. Blood 2005;105(10):3817–23.

3. Sebban C, Mounier N, Brousse N, et al. Standard chemotherapy with interferon compared with CHOP followed by high-dose therapy with autologous stem cell transplantation in untreated patients with advanced follicular lymphoma: the

GELF-94 randomized study from the Groupe d'Etude des Lymphomes de l'Adulte (GELA). Blood 2006;108(8):2540–4.

4. Gyan E, Foussard C, Bertrand P, et al. High-dose therapy followed by autologous purged stem cell transplantation and doxorubicin-based chemotherapy in patients with advanced follicular lymphoma: a randomized multicenter study by the GOELAMS with final results after a median follow-up of 9 years. Blood 2009;113(5):995–1001.

5. Ladetto M, De Marco F, Benedetti F, et al. Prospective, multicenter randomized GITMO/IIL trial comparing intensive (R-HDS) versus conventional (CHOP-R) chemoimmunotherapy in high-risk follicular lymphoma at diagnosis: the superior disease control of R-HDS does not translate into an overall survival advantage. Blood 2008;111(8):4004–13.

6. Schouten HC, Qian W, Kvaloy S, et al. High-dose therapy improves progression-free survival and survival in relapsed follicular non-Hodgkin's lymphoma: results from the randomized European CUP trial. J Clin Oncol 2003;21(21):3918–27.

7. Freedman AS, Neuberg D, Mauch P, et al. Long-term follow-up of autologous bone marrow transplantation in patients with relapsed follicular lymphoma. Blood 1999;94(10):3325–33.

8. Evens AM, Vanderplas A, LaCasce AS, et al. Stem cell transplantation for follicular lymphoma relapsed/refractory after prior rituximab: a comprehensive analysis from the NCCN lymphoma outcomes project. Cancer 2013;119(20):3662–71.

9. Le Gouill S, De Guibert S, Planche L, et al. Impact of the use of autologous stem cell transplantation at first relapse both in naive and previously rituximab exposed follicular lymphoma patients treated in the GELA/GOELAMS FL2000 study. Haematologica 2011;96(8):1128–35.

10. Jiménez-Ubieto A, Grande C, Caballero D, et al. Autologous stem cell transplantation for follicular lymphoma: favorable long-term survival irrespective of pre-transplantation rituximab exposure. Biol Blood Marrow Transplant 2017;23(10): 1631–40.

11. Berinstein NL, Bhella S, Pennell NM, et al. Prolonged clinical remissions in patients with relapsed or refractory follicular lymphoma treated with autologous stem cell transplantation incorporating rituximab. Ann Hematol 2015;94(5): 813–23.

12. Kornacker M, Stumm J, Pott C, et al. Characteristics of relapse after autologous stem-cell transplantation for follicular lymphoma: a long-term follow-up. Ann Oncol 2009;20(4):722–8.

13. Montoto S, Davies AJ, Matthews J, et al. Risk and clinical implications of transformation of follicular lymphoma to diffuse large B-cell lymphoma. J Clin Oncol 2007; 25(17):2426–33.

14. Rohatiner AZ, Nadler L, Davies AJ, et al. Myeloablative therapy with autologous bone marrow transplantation for follicular lymphoma at the time of second or subsequent remission: long-term follow-up. J Clin Oncol 2007;25(18):2554–9.

15. Pettengell R, Uddin R, Boumendil S, et al. Durable benefit of rituximab maintenance postautograft in patients with relapsed follicular lymphoma: 12-year follow-up of the EBMT Lym1 trial. Hematol Oncol 2017;35(S2):32–3.

16. Montoto S, Corradini P, Dreyling M, et al. Indications for hematopoietic stem cell transplantation in patients with follicular lymphoma: a consensus project of the EBMT-Lymphoma Working Party. Haematologica 2013;98(7):1014–21.

17. Dreyling M, Ghielmini M, Rule S, et al. Newly diagnosed and relapsed follicular lymphoma: ESMO clinical practice guidelines for diagnosis, treatment and follow-up. Ann Oncol 2016;27(suppl 5):v83–90.

18. McNamara C, Davies J, Dyer M, et al. Guidelines on the investigation and management of follicular lymphoma. Br J Haematol 2012;156(4):446–67.
19. Tan D, Horning SJ, Hoppe RT, et al. Improvements in observed and relative survival in follicular grade 1-2 lymphoma during 4 decades: the Stanford University experience. Blood 2013;122(6):981–7.
20. Casulo C, Byrtek M, Dawson KL, et al. Early relapse of follicular lymphoma after rituximab plus cyclophosphamide, doxorubicin, vincristine, and prednisone defines patients at high risk for death: an analysis from the national lymphocare study. J Clin Oncol 2015;33(23):2516–22.
21. Federico M, Caballero Barrigón MD, Marcheselli L, et al. Rituximab and the risk of transformation of follicular lymphoma: a retrospective pooled analysis. Lancet Haematol 2018;5(8):e359–67.
22. Jiménez-Ubieto A, Grande C, Caballero D, et al. Autologous stem cell transplantation may be curative for patients with follicular lymphoma with early therapy failure without the need for immunotherapy. Hematol Oncol Stem Cell Ther 2019; 12(4):194–203.
23. Jurinovic V, Metzner B, Pfreundschuh M, et al. Autologous stem cell transplantation for patients with early progression of follicular lymphoma: a follow-up study of 2 randomized trials from the German Low Grade Lymphoma Study Group. Biol Blood Marrow Transplant 2018;24(6):1172–9.
24. Casulo C, Friedberg JW, Ahn KW, et al. Autologous transplantation in follicular lymphoma with early therapy failure: a national lymphocare study and Center for International Blood and Marrow Transplant Research Analysis. Biol Blood Marrow Transplant 2018;24(6):1163–71.
25. Madsen C, Pedersen MB, Vase M, et al. Outcome determinants for transformed indolent lymphomas treated with or without autologous stem-cell transplantation. Ann Oncol 2015;26(2):393–9.
26. Sarkozy C, Trneny M, Xerri L, et al. Risk factors and outcomes for patients with follicular lymphoma who had histologic transformation after response to first-line immunochemotherapy in the PRIMA trial. J Clin Oncol 2016;34(22):2575–82.
27. Godfrey J, Leukam MJ, Smith SM. An update in treating transformed lymphoma. Best Pract Res Clin Haematol 2018;31(3):251–61.
28. Hari P, Carreras J, Zhang MJ, et al. Allogeneic transplants in follicular lymphoma: higher risk of disease progression after reduced-intensity compared to myeloablative conditioning. Biol Blood Marrow Transplant 2008;14(2):236–45.
29. Khouri IF, McLaughlin P, Saliba RM, et al. Eight-year experience with allogeneic stem cell transplantation for relapsed follicular lymphoma after nonmyeloablative conditioning with fludarabine, cyclophosphamide, and rituximab. Blood 2008; 111(12):5530–6.
30. Rezvani AR, Storer B, Maris M, et al. Nonmyeloablative allogeneic hematopoietic cell transplantation in relapsed, refractory, and transformed indolent non-Hodgkin's lymphoma. J Clin Oncol 2008;26(2):211–7.
31. Robinson SP, Goldstone AH, Mackinnon S, et al. Chemoresistant or aggressive lymphoma predicts for a poor outcome following reduced-intensity allogeneic progenitor cell transplantation: an analysis from the Lymphoma Working Party of the European Group for Blood and Bone Marrow Transplantation. Blood 2002;100(13):4310–6.
32. Thomson KJ, Morris EC, Milligan D, et al. T-cell-depleted reduced-intensity transplantation followed by donor leukocyte infusions to promote graft-versus-lymphoma activity results in excellent long-term survival in patients with multiply relapsed follicular lymphoma. J Clin Oncol 2010;28(23):3695–700.

33. Vigouroux S, Michallet M, Porcher R, et al. Long-term outcomes after reduced-intensity conditioning allogeneic stem cell transplantation for low-grade lymphoma: a survey by the French Society of Bone Marrow Graft Transplantation and Cellular Therapy (SFGM-TC). Haematologica 2007;92(5):627–34.

34. Sureda A, Zhang MJ, Dreger P, et al. Allogeneic hematopoietic stem cell transplantation for relapsed follicular lymphoma: a combined analysis on behalf of the Lymphoma Working Party of the EBMT and the Lymphoma Committee of the CIBMTR. Cancer 2018;124(8):1733–42.

35. Robinson SP, Boumendil A, Finel H, et al. Reduced intensity allogeneic stem cell transplantation for follicular lymphoma relapsing after an autologous transplant achieves durable long-term disease control: an analysis from the Lymphoma Working Party of the EBMT†. Ann Oncol 2016;27(6):1088–94.

36. Robinson SP, Canals C, Luang JJ, et al. The outcome of reduced intensity allogeneic stem cell transplantation and autologous stem cell transplantation when performed as a first transplant strategy in relapsed follicular lymphoma: an analysis from the Lymphoma Working Party of the EBMT. Bone Marrow Transplant 2013; 48(11):1409–14.

37. Tomblyn MR, Ewell M, Bredeson C, et al. Autologous versus reduced-intensity allogeneic hematopoietic cell transplantation for patients with chemosensitive follicular non-Hodgkin lymphoma beyond first complete response or first partial response. Biol Blood Marrow Transplant 2011;17(7):1051–7.

38. Wirk B, Fenske TS, Hamadani M, et al. Outcomes of hematopoietic cell transplantation for diffuse large B cell lymphoma transformed from follicular lymphoma. Biol Blood Marrow Transplant 2014;20(7):951–9.

39. Smith SM, Godfrey J, Ahn KW, et al. Autologous transplantation versus allogeneic transplantation in patients with follicular lymphoma experiencing early treatment failure. Cancer 2018;124(12):2541–51.

40. El-Najjar I, Boumendil A, Luan JJ, et al. The impact of total body irradiation on the outcome of patients with follicular lymphoma treated with autologous stem-cell transplantation in the modern era: a retrospective study of the EBMT Lymphoma Working Party. Ann Oncol 2014;25(11):2224–9.

41. Montoto S, Canals C, Rohatiner AZ, et al. Long-term follow-up of high-dose treatment with autologous haematopoietic progenitor cell support in 693 patients with follicular lymphoma: an EBMT registry study. Leukemia 2007;21(11):2324–31.

42. Jiménez-Ubieto A, Grande C, Caballero D, et al. Secondary malignancies and survival outcomes after autologous stem cell transplantation for follicular lymphoma in the pre-rituximab and rituximab eras: a long-term follow-up analysis from the Spanish GELTAMO registry. Bone Marrow Transplant 2018;53(6):780–3.

43. Genovese G, Kähler AK, Handsaker RE, et al. Clonal hematopoiesis and blood-cancer risk inferred from blood DNA sequence. N Engl J Med 2014;371(26): 2477–87.

44. Jaiswal S, Fontanillas P, Flannick J, et al. Age-related clonal hematopoiesis associated with adverse outcomes. N Engl J Med 2014;371(26):2488–98.

45. Jaiswal S, Natarajan P, Silver AJ, et al. Clonal hematopoiesis and risk of atherosclerotic cardiovascular disease. N Engl J Med 2017;377(2):111–21.

46. Acuna-Hidalgo R, Sengul H, Steehouwer M, et al. Ultra-sensitive sequencing identifies high prevalence of clonal hematopoiesis-associated mutations throughout adult life. Am J Hum Genet 2017;101(1):50–64.

47. Abelson S, Collord G, Ng SWK, et al. Prediction of acute myeloid leukaemia risk in healthy individuals. Nature 2018;559(7714):400–4.

48. Gibson CJ, Lindsley RC, Tchekmedyian V, et al. Clonal hematopoiesis associated with adverse outcomes after autologous stem-cell transplantation for lymphoma. J Clin Oncol 2017;35(14):1598–605.

49. Frick M, Chan W, Arends CM, et al. Role of donor clonal hematopoiesis in allogeneic hematopoietic stem-cell transplantation. J Clin Oncol 2019;37(5):375–85.

50. Wong TN, Miller CA, Jotte MRM, et al. Cellular stressors contribute to the expansion of hematopoietic clones of varying leukemic potential. Nat Commun 2018; 9(1):455.

51. Ortmann CA, Dorsheimer L, Abou-El-Ardat K, et al. Functional dominance of CHIP-mutated hematopoietic stem cells in patients undergoing autologous transplantation. Cell Rep 2019;27(7):2022–8.e3.

52. Jensen MC, Popplewell L, Cooper LJ, et al. Antitransgene rejection responses contribute to attenuated persistence of adoptively transferred CD20/CD19-specific chimeric antigen receptor redirected T cells in humans. Biol Blood Marrow Transplant 2010;16(9):1245–56.

53. Kochenderfer JN, Wilson WH, Janik JE, et al. Eradication of B-lineage cells and regression of lymphoma in a patient treated with autologous T cells genetically engineered to recognize CD19. Blood 2010;116(20):4099–102.

54. Schuster SJ, Svoboda J, Chong EA, et al. Chimeric antigen receptor T cells in refractory B-cell lymphomas. N Engl J Med 2017;377(26):2545–54.

55. Schuster SJ, Bishop MR, Tam CS, et al. Tisagenlecleucel in adult relapsed or refractory diffuse large B-cell lymphoma. N Engl J Med 2019;380(1):45–56.

56. Neelapu SS, Tummala S, Kebriaei P, et al. Chimeric antigen receptor T-cell therapy - assessment and management of toxicities. Nat Rev Clin Oncol 2018;15(1): 47–62.

57. Hirayama AV, Gauthier J, Hay KA, et al. High rate of durable complete remission in follicular lymphoma after CD19 CAR-T cell immunotherapy. Blood 2019;134(7): 636–40.

58. Neelapu SS, Locke FL, Bartlett NL, et al. Axicabtagene ciloleucel CAR T-cell therapy in refractory large B-cell lymphoma. N Engl J Med 2017;377(26):2531–44.

59. Lee DW, Santomasso BD, Locke FL, et al. ASTCT consensus grading for cytokine release syndrome and neurologic toxicity associated with immune effector cells. Biol Blood Marrow Transplant 2019;25(4):625–38.

60. Till BG, Jensen MC, Wang J, et al. CD20-specific adoptive immunotherapy for lymphoma using a chimeric antigen receptor with both CD28 and 4-1BB domains: pilot clinical trial results. Blood 2012;119(17):3940–50.

61. Qin H, Ramakrishna S, Nguyen S, et al. Preclinical development of bivalent chimeric antigen receptors targeting both CD19 and CD22. Mol Ther Oncolytics 2018;11:127–37.

62. Curran KJ, Seinstra BA, Nikhamin Y, et al. Enhancing antitumor efficacy of chimeric antigen receptor T cells through constitutive CD40L expression. Mol Ther 2015;23(4):769–78.

63. Dafni U, Michielin O, Lluesma SM, et al. Efficacy of adoptive therapy with tumor-infiltrating lymphocytes and recombinant interleukin-2 in advanced cutaneous melanoma: a systematic review and meta-analysis. Ann Oncol 2019;30(12): 1902–13.

64. Zacharakis N, Chinnasamy H, Black M, et al. Immune recognition of somatic mutations leading to complete durable regression in metastatic breast cancer. Nat Med 2018;24(6):724–30.

65. Matasar MJ, Luminari S, Barr PM, et al. Follicular lymphoma: recent and emerging therapies, treatment strategies, and remaining unmet needs. Oncologist 2019;24(11):e1236–50.
66. Solal-Céligny P, Roy P, Colombat P, et al. Follicular lymphoma international prognostic index. Blood 2004;104(5):1258–65.
67. Federico M, Bellei M, Marcheselli L, et al. Follicular lymphoma international prognostic index 2: a new prognostic index for follicular lymphoma developed by the international follicular lymphoma prognostic factor project. J Clin Oncol 2009; 27(27):4555–62.
68. Bachy E, Maurer MJ, Habermann TM, et al. A simplified scoring system in de novo follicular lymphoma treated initially with immunochemotherapy. Blood 2018;132(1):49–58.
69. Okosun J, Bödör C, Wang J, et al. Integrated genomic analysis identifies recurrent mutations and evolution patterns driving the initiation and progression of follicular lymphoma. Nat Genet 2014;46(2):176–81.
70. Green MR, Kihira S, Liu CL, et al. Mutations in early follicular lymphoma progenitors are associated with suppressed antigen presentation. Proc Natl Acad Sci U S A 2015;112(10):E1116–25.
71. Kridel R, Chan FC, Mottok A, et al. Histological transformation and progression in follicular lymphoma: a clonal evolution study. PLoS Med 2016;13(12):e1002197.

Immunomodulatory Agents in Follicular Lymphoma

Loic Ysebaert, MD, PhD[a], Franck Morschhauser, MD, PhD[b],*

KEYWORDS

- Chemo-free approaches • Follicular lymphoma • Immunomodulatory agents
- Monoclonal antibodies • Tumor immune microenvironment

KEY POINTS

- Immunomodulatory agents are now part of modern follicular lymphoma therapeutic management.
- They offer a chemo-free strategy that provides a clinical benefit even for high-risk disease.
- These strategies target tumor cells both directly and through microenvironment modifications.
- We are still lacking biomarkers predicting efficacy of immunomodulatory agents.

INTRODUCTION

Thinking about the mechanisms that establish the need for immune-mediated targeting with follicular lymphoma (FL) therapies, the term "immune rheostat" comes to mind. In an electric circuit, a rheostat is an adjustable resistor for regulating a current by means of variable resistance, used to fine-tune the throttle of a motor, for example. So, in the tumor microenvironment, we define the immune rheostat as the instrument used to control FL outgrowth (not a current) by varying the resistance applied to cancer cells, to avoid their immune escape (**Fig. 1**).

GENOMICS IN FOLLICULAR LYMPHOMA: SWITCHING OFF THE IMMUNE RHEOSTAT

FL is the paradigm of a germinal center (GC)-derived cancer with recurrent somatic mutations, but with respect to architectural constraints is in opposition to GC-derived diffuse large B-cell lymphoma (DLBCL).[1–3] Recent evidence demonstrates that most of the recurrent mutations also dictate how cancer cells shape their supportive niches for autonomous survival, by excluding potential harmful neighbors.[1,4]

[a] Service d'Hematologie, Institut Universitaire du Cancer de Toulouse-Oncopole, Center for Cancer Research of Toulouse (CRCT), Inserm UMR1037, IUC-Toulouse-Oncopole, 1 Avenue Irene Joliot-Curie, Toulouse 31059, France; [b] Univ. Lille, CHU Lille, ULR 7365 - GRITA - Groupe de Recherche Sur les Formes Injectables et les Technologies Associees, Lille F-59000, France
* Corresponding author.
E-mail address: franck.morschhauser@chru-lille.fr

Hematol Oncol Clin N Am 34 (2020) 715–726
https://doi.org/10.1016/j.hoc.2020.02.007

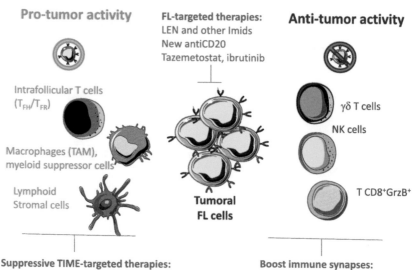

Fig. 1. Protumoral and antitumoral activities of the immune microenvironment of follicular lymphoma, and how to target it. IDO, indoleamine 2,3 oxidase; T_{FH}/T_{FR}, T follicular helper/regulatory.

A recent whole exome and transcriptome sequencing study[5] in 1042 cases revealed that FL cells demonstrate a significant degree of genetic heterogeneity (with more than 100 genes mutated with a frequency of at least 2%), but that nearly 100% of cases had a mutation in at least one chromatin-modifying gene (the most frequently mutated genes being *KMT2D* [lysine methyltransferase 2D], *BCL2* [B-cell lymphoma 2], *IGLL5* [immunoglobulin lambda-like polypeptide 5] and *CREBBP* [cAMP-response element binding protein]), as previously reported.[6–8] Transcriptome analysis indicated a strong correlation between mutations in the antiapoptotic, ubiquitin-conjugating enzyme BIRC6 (baculoviral IAP repeat-containing protein 6), and the pattern of immune infiltration (enriched in "macrophage genes"). Disruption of *KMT2D* perturbs GC B-cell development and promotes lymphomagenesis, and the *CREBBP* acetyltransferase is a haplo-insufficient tumor suppressor in FL.[7,8] Moreover, somatic mutations altering *EZH2* (on the tyrosine 641 residue) in 15% of patients with FL have been recognized since 2010 to be involved in repressing global gene expression through methylation.[9] Functional consequences of histone acetylation-regulating gene *CREBBP* "loss-of-function" mutations include impaired p53 activation (while promoting oncogenic *Bcl-6* repressor gene effects), blocking exit from the germinal center. On the other hand, consequences of "gain-of-function" mutations in the catalytic domain of polycomb repressor complex-2 (PRC-2), enhancer of zeste homolog 2 (EZH2) enzyme, are the improvement of efficient trimethylation of histones (H3K27me), proliferation, and differentiation blockade.[10] A second hit is nonetheless needed for full-blown lymphomatous disease to install in mice models, as exemplified by *EZH2* mutations cooperating with *Bcl-2* deregulation.[11]

Single-agent studies of epigenetic-modifying agents have pinpointed the need to develop efficient combinations, and those using immunotherapy hold real promise.[10]

Immune escape from tumor infiltrating lymphocytes (TILs) is a hallmark of cancers, including FL.[12] The frequency of perturbed antigen presentation to natural killer (NK) or T cells machinery is high in GC B-cell–derived lymphomas.[13,14] In DLBCL, *EZH2* mutations are linked to the loss of major histocompatibility complex (MHC) class I and II expression (and reduced TILs infiltration).[14] In FL, MHC class I expression is reduced thanks to beta2-microglobulin (*β2M*) gene mutations (destabilizing MHC protein at the cellular surface), and MHC class II expression is dampened by CREB-binding protein mutations (60% of patients), avoiding recognition by CD4+ and CD8+ T cells. Another frequent somatic mutation leading to tumor necrosis factor receptor superfamily 14/herpesvirus entry mediator (TNFRSF14/HVEM) loss-of-function (found in 50% of FL patients) alleviates the inhibitory effect of its interaction with B and T lymphocyte attenuator (BTLA), and triggers an amplification of BTLA^hi-follicular helper T cells (Tfh) and subsequent secretion of FL soluble factors, which then activates the FL-cancer-associated fibroblasts (FL-CAFs) to set up a dedicated niche.[15] As a consequence, FL-CAFs express discrete sets of surface receptors and/or ligands, and secrete soluble factors, to enhance the following:

i. Interactions of FL cells with CD4+ Tfh cells
ii. B-cell activation and retention
iii. Recruitment of circulating myeloid cells to support myeloid-derived suppressor cells/tumor associated macrophages (MDSC/TAM) differentiation, blocking T and NK responses (secretion of prostaglandin E2)

CONSEQUENCES OF THE PERTURBED IMMUNE RHEOSTAT: LOSS OF IMMUNE SYNAPSE

The very first attempts of delineating immune infiltration in FL were based on tumor "bulk analysis" by deconvolution of transcriptomes. Dave and colleagues[16] (in 2004) pioneered the studies linking the nature of transcriptomic signatures of nonmalignant immune cells (immune response 1 enriched in T cells and immune response 2 enriched in macrophages/dendritic cells) and prognosis. In 2009, the dysfunction of T-cell immunologic synapse (and its repair with lenalidomide [LEN]) in FL was unraveled, linking intrafollicular expression of a cytolytic effector molecule (here Rab27A) with prognosis.[17] Importantly, these problems in CD4+ and CD8+ T-cell "kiss of death" responses are actively induced by direct contacts with FL cells and transferable to allogeneic, healthy T cells. They are not seen in peripheral T cells lacking tumor interactions, and thus are not a consequence of a patient's intrinsic immune cell defects.[17,18] The problem resides in the adequate polarization of granules, an event that is impossible to detect with transcriptome analyses. Treatment of both T and B cells with LEN restores adequate F-actin polymerization, tyrosine phosphorylation events, and cell killing irrespectively of the presence of exogenous antigen. After 2010, other studies investigated the localization and functionality of CD8+ T and NK cells interspersed in the interfollicular spaces, and linked cytotoxic capacities (based on gene signatures and granzyme B expression), to prognosis after R-CHOP (rituximab, cyclophosphamide, doxorubicin, vincristine, and prednisone).[19,20] Yet, a stringent statistical analysis of immunohistochemistry (IHC) stainings and transcriptomes of the TILs (CD3, CD4, CD8, PD-1 [programmed death-1], FOXP3 [forkhead box P3], and ICOS [inducible costimulatory]) from patients enrolled in the PRIMA clinical trial failed to predict progression-free survival (PFS) in the rituximab (RTX) maintenance arm.[19] To increase further complexity, the most recent single-cell sequencing studies of diverse FL-involved sites in 5 patients showed that T cells also had distinct functional states. In regulatory and T follicular helper cells, both activated and putative resting clusters were identified, whereas in effector T cells, cytotoxic (enriched in granzyme A and B) and exhausted (enriched in TIGIT [T-cell immunoreceptor with immunoglobulin and immunoreceptor tyrosine-based inhibitory motif domain], CXCL13 [chemokine (C-X-C motif) ligand 3], LAG3 [lymphocyte-activation gene 3]) clusters were identified based on tumor sites.[21] Expression of parallel transcriptomes in thousands of tumor cells and TILs (at the single-cell level) will foster the development of a systems-level view of the tumor microenvironment.[22]

HEATING UP THE RHEOSTAT IN FOLLICULAR LYMPHOMA: OVERRIDE THE INHIBITORY CHECKPOINTS

Impairment of T-cell synapses by blocking phospho-tyrosine events downstream of T-cell receptor is mediated by immune checkpoint inhibitory receptors (IRs) and their ligands on antigen-presenting cells (including the tumor itself, but also bystander cells in the tumor immune microenvironment [TIME]).[23–26] On ligation, IRs induce apoptosis, anergy, or functional exhaustion of the $\alpha\beta$ T/NK/$\gamma\delta$ T cells involved. In the FL TIME, IR/ligands pairs are manifold.[27] Immune escape may involve the interaction of PD-1 receptor (CD279) with its ligand programmed death-ligand-1 (PD-L1) or PD-L2, or of cytotoxic T-lymphocyte-associated antigen-4 (CTLA-4) with its ligands CD80/CD86 (to which it binds with higher affinity than the costimulatory CD28 molecule), the most eminent regulators of the immune checkpoints against pathogens or cancer cells. It may also implicate a cooperation between CTLA-4/PD-1 and LAG-3 (CD223, lymphocyte-activation gene-3, interacting with MHC-II [better than CD-4], galectin 3), TIM-3 (CD366, T-cell immunoglobulin-containing and mucin-domain-containing molecule 3, interacting with galectin-9, phosphatidylserines, HMGB1), TIGIT, and/or some B7 family of receptors (other than CD80/CD86 and PD-L1/L2: B7-H3, B7-H4, B7-H5, VISTA [V-domain immunoglobulin suppressor of T-cell activation]). FL cells do not express PD-L1, but myeloid cells do in 20% to 30% of cases. TIGIT ligands CD122 and CD155 are expressed by endothelial and dendritic cells, and CD161 (an NK-specific IR)-ligands are found on FL cells. Immunosuppressive regulatory T cells/regulatory follicular T (Treg/Tfr) cells, MDSC cells, and TAMs may also express IR-ligands, and thus reduce the efficacy of innate and adaptive immune cell responses. Last, on those cell-cell contacts, secretion of CCL22, interleukin (IL)-10, arginase 1 and indoleamine 2,3-dioxygenase (IDO) permits local T-cell blockade, but also recruitment of new myeloid and lymphoid cells from the bloodstream to the tumor bed, and their further differentiation into suppressive TAMs, MDSCs, or regulatory T cells (reviewed in Refs.[1–3]).

Overriding the ability of FL cells to evade immune synapses and establish multiple immune inhibitory checkpoints, together with eliciting new synapses (either synthetic, or with available immune cells within the TIME), are the objectives of immunomodulating agents in FL.

IntIMiDation OF FOLLICULAR LYMPHOMA CELLS: MECHANISMS OF ACTION OF LENALIDOMIDE

LEN belongs to the immunomodulatory family of drugs (IMiDs). The direct target of LEN is the ubiquitously expressed E3 ubiquitin-ligase cereblon, inducing ubiquitination and degradation of many targets, including transcription factors (IRF-4, Aiolos, Ikaros).[28] In FL cells, those degradations lead to an increase of interferon (IFN)-responsive genes expression and apoptosis, but in T cells, results in enhanced costimulation signaling and increased IL-2 secretion. Furthermore, in vitro and in vivo analyses showed that LEN harnesses a vast array of antitumoral effects, including

IR-ligand modulation (upregulation of CD80/CD86, CD1c, CD40, and downregulation of PD-L1), rendering cells more visible to surrounding normal immune effector cells (a "tumor-flare" effect is even seen sometimes in patients the first days of LEN treatment). In the TIME, LEN also increased cell numbers and functionality of T, NK, $\gamma\delta$ T, and dendritic cells, and promoted the restoration of an effective immune synapse.[17,28,29] LEN (25 mg/d d1-21/28, 12 cycles) was initially evaluated in 43 patients with indolent non-Hodgkin lymphoma (NHL), including 22 patients with FL in the pilot NHL-001 study, yielding 27% overall response rate (ORR) and 9% complete response (CR), and a median PFS of 4.4 months.[30] In the 19 FL grade 3 patients recruited in the NHL-003 study, ORR/CR rates were slightly improved at 42%/11%, with a median PFS of 8.9 months.[31]

LEN monotherapy thus induced encouraging response rates, but not long-lasting. These first data nonetheless paved the way for association with tolerable agents inducing prolonged responses, namely the anti-CD20 monoclonal antibodies.

TWO-HIT COUNTERSTRIKE AGAINST FOLLICULAR LYMPHOMA CELLS: RATIONALE FOR LENALIDOMIDE + antiCD20 COMBINATIONS
Lenalidomide + Rituximab: the First Chemo-Free Doublet Approved in Follicular Lymphoma

The rationale for increased efficacy with RTX (class I antibody) or obinutuzumab (OBZ, class II antibody) with enhanced antibody-dependent cell-mediated cytotoxicity (ADCC, mediated by CD16+ NK or $\gamma\delta$ T cells) and phagocytosis (ADCP, mediated by CD16+ TAMs) is supported by the increase of NK cell numbers with increased IFNγ and perforin secretion, without down-modulation of the CD20 molecule at the surface of target lymphoma cells.[28] In various clinical trials, LEN + RTX showed synergy in terms of ORR, but also reactivated dysfunctional T/NK cells, improving proliferation and RTX-mediated ADCC in an ancillary study.[32] These results were rapidly confirmed in RTX-LEN combination trials. The SAKK 35/10 study of RTX alone or with LEN in frontline patients reported a respective CR/unconfirmed CR (CRu) rate of 25% versus 36%, with median PFS of 2.3 versus 5.0 years.[33] With a lenalidomide dose of 20 mg/d d1-21/28 combined with standard dose RTX (responders after 6 cycles could continue for 12 cycles) for up to 12 cycles, the MD Anderson Cancer Center phase II study in frontline patients with FL, ORR/CR rates in FL were 98%/76% and estimated 3-year PFS was 79%, independent from FL International Prognostic Index score or tumor bulk.[34] Based on these first trials, the phase III "RELEVANCE" trial randomized 1053 patients requiring therapy according to Groupe d'Etude des Lymphomes Folliculaires (GELF) criteria, between R-chemo and LEN + RTX.[35] At 120 weeks, the Independent Review Committee (IRC)-assessed ORR/CR rates (65%/53% vs 61%/48%) and estimated 3-year PFS (78% vs 77%) were reported for for R-chemo and LEN + RTX groups, respectively. The 3-year overall survival (OS; 94% in both arms) was very comparable for R-chemo and LEN + RTX arms, respectively.[35] Skin toxicities were more frequently observed in the chemo-free LEN + RTX arm, and neutropenia was more frequent in the R-chemo arm.

In the relapsed setting, the phase III AUGMENT trial recently confirmed in 295 patients with FL that LEN + RTX improved PFS (OS results are still maturing) versus RTX-placebo, with IRC-assessed ORR/CR rates of 80%/35% versus 55%/20% in the control arm, and median PFS was 39.4 versus 13.9 months, respectively,[36] confirming phase II trial results.[37,38] Neutropenia was the most common grade 3/4 event, but easily manageable. These encouraging results were reproduced in an interim report of the phase III MAGNIFY trial in patients with relapsed/refractory (R/R) FL (n = 296), randomizing patients to RTX or LEN + RTX maintenance until progression after 12 months LEN + RTX induction; ORR/CR rates were 74%/46%, and median PFS was 30.2 months.[39] Food and Drug Administration approval and positive European Medicines Agency opinion (https://www.ema.europa.eu/en/documents/smop/chmp-post-authorisation-summary-positive-opinion-revlimid-ii-107_en.pdf) were supported by the AUGMENT and MAGNIFY results for previously treated patients with FL to receive up to 12 cycles of LEN in combination with an RTX product.

Lenalidomide + Obinutuzumab: Another Promising Chemo-Free Backbone in Follicular Lymphoma

OBZ has been developed as an ADCC/ADCP super inducer antibody, but also binds differently to its CD20 epitopes, inducing direct cell killing.[40,41] In vitro analyses of 3-dimensional spheroids (from FL cell lines) have also highlighted its higher ability to activate CD16-mediated NK and $\gamma\delta$ T cytotoxicity, but also to interfere with kinase intracellular cascades, leading to lysosomal cell death and senescence of tumor cells.[42] OBZ single agent versus RTX single agent (induction + maintenance) has been evaluated in the randomized phase II GAUSS study.[43] ORR and CR/CRu assessed by investigators in the FL cohort were 45% and 12% in the OBZ arm compared with 33% and 5% in the RTX arm after the induction period (66%/42% vs 64%/23% during the entire treatment period including induction and maintenance), suggesting that OBZ may induce deeper responses. OBZ also yielded a higher rate of MRD-negative responses, translating into a significantly prolonged PFS, in the GADO-LIN and GALLIUM phase III trials in combination to chemotherapy.[44,45] Similar to LEN + RTX trials, LEN + OBZ has also been investigated in the context of phase II studies in France, using LEN 20 mg d1-21/28 six cycles + OBZ 1000 mg each month as an induction phase, followed by a maintenance phase with LEN 10 mg for 12 cycles, with OBZ every 2 months for 2 years.[46] In the frontline setting, according to 2007 International Working Group criteria, ORR/CR rates were as high as 96%/59%, 85% having a complete metabolic response (using the Deauville 5 points scale of 1–3).[47] Two-year estimates for PFS (85%) and also OS (97%) confirmed that LEN + OBZ was highly active in untreated FL. In the relapsed/refractory setting, ORR/CR rates in 86 evaluable patients (28% of whom had progressed before 2 years after their last therapy) were 79%/38%, with an estimated 2-year PFS of 67%.[47] These PFS rates were comparable to autologous stem cell transplantation strategies.

Frontline antiCD20+LEN in patients with FL was shown to be at least as effective as the most effective chemoimmunotherapy (CIT) regimens (even with OBZ), which have a projected 10-year OS of 81%, and 30 month-CR rate of 53%.[35] To avoid early relapse (16% of POD24 in patients receiving LEN + RTX in the RELEVANCE trial, 9% of POD24 in the GALLIUM trial[45]), one should now consider combining antiCD20+LEN + a third drug with a specific mechanism of action, without increasing toxicity.

BUILDING ON LENALIDOMIDE + antiCD20 CHEMO-FREE BACKBONE: TARGETING IMMUNE CHECKPOINTS

Scarce data have been presented with nivolumab and pembrolizumab in the treatment of R/R FL, and will be developed by others in this journal. PD-L1 targeting with atezolizumab, to improve the safety profile in terms of immune-related adverse events, in combination with LEN + OBZ (6 months induction, and 24 months maintenance) yielded ORR/CR rates of 78%/72%, and a 12-month PFS of 77.5%.[48] Interestingly, 15 of 16 CR patients also had undetectable minimal residual disease (MRD), translating into an improvement of PFS.

PD-1/PD-L1 axis is not the only checkpoint raised by tumor cells against immune effector cell recognition. Because LEN improves cell killing induced by antiCD20 antibodies, it may also be useful in the improvement of another inhibitory checkpoint, between TAMs and FL cells this time. Blockade of CD47/SIRPα immune checkpoint (CD47 is a "don't eat me" signal opposed to macrophages by tumor cells to evade phagocytosis) is also of interest.[49] In a phase Ib/II trial, an anti-CD47 IgG4 (to restrict Fc receptor engagement) antibody in combination with RTX induces ORR/CR rates of 71%/43%, with most of the responders still relapse-free after more than 8 months of follow-up. The phase II has started to recruit, and first results presented in the R/R FL cohort show ORR/CR rates of 61%/24%.[50] In FL biopsies, recent work highlighted that TAMs have various degrees of CD14 and signal-regulating protein alpha (SIRPα) expression levels, underpinning their functionalities.[51] On one hand, CD14$^+$SIRPα^{hi} macrophages exhibit TAMs differentiation markers (CD163+, CD117+, really close to nurselike cells [NLC], the M2-TAMs in patients with chronic lymphocytic leukemia), and are able to phagocytose target cells (even more with RTX), and also suppress T-cell function. In this study, this subset was associated with inferior outcomes.[51] On the other hand, CD14$^-$SIRPα^{neg} macrophages stimulate T-cell function, and phagocytose with less efficiency. Interestingly, those data are aligned with CLL studies, showing that LEN reduces pronurturing functions of NLCs, which acquire properties of phagocytosis, and promote T-cell proliferation together with a loss of M2 markers like CD163 and a skewing toward an M1-like differentiation program.[52] We do not know the effects of LEN on CD47/SIRPα expressions, but because a second pro-phagocytic signal, combined with the blockade of CD47/SIRPα interactions, is mandatory to enhance the clearance of tumor cells through ADCP, LEN is a good candidate drug in a triplet.

Costimulatory molecules on T cells, such as 4-1BB (CD137), ICOS, CD27, and OX40, can be leveraged for FL immunotherapy.[53] CD137 (4-1BB) is a surface protein on activated T lymphocytes (intrafollicular CD4+ T cells in FL),[54] but also activated NK cells, B cells, and myeloid cells, including mature dendritic cells in the TIME. Urelumab is an agonist antibody to CD137, evaluated in 346 patients with cancer.[55] Above 1 mg/kg dose, severe transaminitis can occur, with induction of IFN-response genes and cytokines related to T-cell activation. Further clinical development is hampered by both dependency on Fcγ receptor-mediated hyperclustering and hepatotoxicity.[56] Combination with LEN may be detrimental for the safety profile of this antibody. Yet, recent advances pinpointed that better activity and tolerance of CD137 therapeutic antibodies depend on their isotype and intrinsic agonist strength. All FcγRs can crosslink anti-CD137, but to increase efficacy, we must work on engineering the CD137 targeting antibodies to avoid liver toxicity.

These 3 options are thought to increase the efficacy of "natural" immune synapses, primed by LEN, together with a blockade of the inhibitory (or stimulation of an activating) second signal. Another avenue for drug development relies on the induction of "synthetic" synapses, to an extent that is usually not seen in patients, thanks to chimeric antigen receptor (CAR)-T cells or bispecific antibodies.

A GLIMPSE INTO THE FUTURE: IMPROVING "SYNTHETIC" IMMUNE SYNAPSES WITH LENALIDOMIDE

With accumulating data proving the efficacy of IMiDS in the restoration of immune synapses, there is no doubt that LEN should be considered to intensify CAR cell therapy[57] and/or bispecific antibodies (bs-Abs)-induced killing. Bispecific antibodies carry an Fc fragment devoid of Fc receptor–binding moieties, allowing drug dosing every week or up to 3 weeks. Bispecific antibodies couple T cells and FL cells to form a lytic synapse, that resembles the mechanism of T-cell receptor (TCR)-peptide MHC interactions[58]; the difference is the larger size and number of synapses. Depending on expression levels of tumor targets (CD20, CD47, CD137), those antibodies in theory may establish 50 to 100,000 contacts (T-cell activation through MHC-peptide starts at 10 contacts).

Mosunetuzumab is a full-length CD20/CD3 T-dependent bispecific antibody. The phase I trial (GO29781) yielded ORR/CR rates of 61%/50% in 18 evaluable relapsed FL patients.[59] Another CD3/CD20 T-cell bispecific antibody (CD20-TCB; with a 2:1 molecular format, binding to molecules of CD20 and one of CD3) called RG6026 was infused every 2 weeks then 3 weeks in 18 patients with FL (and 20 transformed FL) of 98 patients with B-cell lymphoma.[60] In the 10-mg cohort, CD20-TCB induced 57% ORR/26% CR rates. With both agents, grade 3/4 reporting suggests a very good safety profile: 0% cytokine release syndrome (CRS), 3% neurologic, and 20% neutropenia (3% febrile), with only 3% leading to drug discontinuation. Extending these first results, REGN1979 CD3xCD20 bs-Ab infused every week for 3 months, then every other week for 6 other months, in 21 patients with transformed or refractory FL at doses greater than 5 mg resulted in unprecedented ORR/CR rates of 93%/71%.[61]

To mitigate those side effects, step-up dosing regimens are needed, and infusion of OBZ (to decrease normal B-cell counts, T-cell activation, and subsequently cytokine release, in the peripheral blood) before bs-Ab ramp-up is often indicated.[62] Activity of bs-Abs may rely on target motility, and the distance between epitope and the target membrane. Trivalent 1 + 2 designs exist, which afford increased antigen avidity, T-cell activation, and cell killing. If the tumor target is expressed by many normal cells (eg, CD47, at the surface of red blood cells), the development of CD19xCD47 bs-Abs allows for increased CD47-mediated phagocytosis of CD19+ target cells,[63] inhibits BCR signaling to a higher extent than a CD19 mAb,[64] and retains its activity in the presence of high amounts of non–tumor-associated CD47. The issue of CD137-triggered FcγR clustering and hepatotoxicity, trimeric CD137xCD19 bs-Abs have been developed, and used in association with antiCD20-TCB in mice models. Indeed, the latter bs-Abs increased CD137 at the surface of CD8+ T cells, so the former triggered a second activation of effector cells.[65]

Because bs-Abs are "off-the-shelf," ready-to-use drugs, and do not need any T-cell manipulation, they will challenge CAR-T cells in the therapy of refractory B-cell indolent lymphomas.

SUMMARY

Immunomodulating agents restoring the immune rheostat and controlling the progression of FL carry great promise. LEN recently confirmed in the context of large, controlled randomized trials, its efficacy and good tolerance. IMiDs are destined to become important building blocks for combinatorial strategies with monoclonal antibodies (including OBZ), novel targeted immune checkpoint blockers (eg, atezolizumab, anti-CD47), and emerging cellular immunotherapies to elicit strong and long-lasting immune synapses. Yet, we are still lacking both treatment-specific and disease-specific biomarkers to promote the use of chemo-free approaches in frontline patients with FL.

DISCLOSURE

F. Morschhauser: Consultancy (F. Hoffmann-La Roche), honoraria for scientific lectures (Celgene, F. Hoffmann-La Roche, and Janssen), Advisory committee (Bayer, Bristol-Myers Squibb, Celgene, Epizyme, F. Hoffmann-La Roche, and Gilead). L.

Ysebaert: Consultancy (AbbVie, F. Hoffmann-La Roche, Gilead, and Janssen), honoraria for scientific lectures (AbbVie, Astra-Zeneca, Celgene, F. Hoffmann-La Roche, Gilead, Janssen).

REFERENCES

1. Scott DW, Gascoyne RD. The tumour microenvironment in B-cell lymphomas. Nat Rev Cancer 2014;14:517–34.
2. Tarte K. Role of the microenvironment across histological subtypes of NHL. Hematology Am Soc Hematol Educ Program 2017;2017(1):610–7.
3. Verdiere L, Mourcin F, Tarte K. Microenvironment signaling driving lymphomagenesis. Curr Opin Hematol 2018;25:335–45.
4. Huet S, Sujobert P, Salles G. From genetics to the clinic: a translational perspective on follicular lymphoma. Nat Rev Cancer 2018;18:224–39.
5. Li X, Kositsky R, Anupama Reddy A, et al. Whole exome and transcriptome sequencing in 1042 cases reveals distinct clinically relevant genetic subgroups of follicular lymphoma. American Society of Hematology meeting 2019, abstract #19. Orlando, December 7-10, 2019.
6. Morin RD, Mendez-Lago M, Mungall AJ, et al. Frequent mutation of histone-modifying genes in non-Hodgkin lymphoma. Nature 2011;476:298–303.
7. Zhang J, Dominguez-Sola D, Hussein S, et al. Disruption of KMT2D perturbs germinal center B cell development and promotes lymphomagenesis. Nat Med 2015;21:1190–8.
8. Zhang J, Vlasevska S, Wells VA, et al. The CREBBP acetyltransferase is a haploinsufficient tumor suppressor in B-cell lymphoma. Cancer Discov 2017;7: 322–37.
9. McCabe MT, Ott HM, Ganji G, et al. EZH2 inhibition as a therapeutic strategy for lymphoma with EZH2-activated mutations. Nature 2012;492:108–14.
10. Sermer D, Pasqualucci L, Wendel HG, et al. Emerging epigenetic-modulating therapies in lymphoma. Nat Rev Clin Oncol 2019;16:494–507.
11. Berg T, Thoene S, Yap D, et al. A transgenic mouse model demonstrating the oncogenic role of mutations in the polycomb-group gene EZH2 in lymphomagenesis. Blood 2014;123:3914–24.
12. Hanahan D, Weinberg RA. Hallmarks of cancer: the next generation. Cell 2011; 144:646–74.
13. Challa-Malladi M, Lieu YK, Califano O, et al. Combined genetic inactivation of beta2-microglobulin and CD58 reveals frequent escape from immune recognition in diffuse large B cell lymphoma. Cancer Cell 2011;20:728–40.
14. Ennishi D, Takata K, Béguelin W, et al. Molecular and genetic characterization of MHC deficiency identifies EZH2 as therapeutic target for enhancing immune recognition. Cancer Discov 2019;9:546–63.
15. Boice M, Salloum D, Mourcin F, et al. Loss of the HVEM tumor suppressor in lymphoma and restoration by modified CAR-T cells. Cell 2016;167:405–18.
16. Dave SS, Wright G, Tan B, et al. Prediction of survival in follicular lymphoma based on molecular features of tumor-infiltrating immune cells. N Engl J Med 2004;351:2159–69.
17. Ramsay AG, Clear AJ, Kelly G, et al. Follicular lymphoma cells induce T-cell immunologic synapse dysfunction that can be repaired with lenalidomide: implications for the tumor microenvironment and immunotherapy. Blood 2009;114: 4713–20.

18. Kiaii S, Clear AJ, Ramsay AG, et al. Follicular lymphoma cells induce changes in T-cell gene expression and function: potential impact on survival and risk of transformation. J Clin Oncol 2013;31:2654–61.

19. Xerri L, Huet S, Venstrom JM, et al. Rituximab treatment circumvents the prognostic impact of tumor-infiltrating T-cells in follicular lymphoma patients. Hum Pathol 2017;64:128–36.

20. Laurent C, Müller S, Do C, et al. Distribution, function, and prognostic value of cytotoxic T lymphocytes in follicular lymphoma: a 3-D tissue-imaging study. Blood 2011;118:5371–9.

21. Haebe S, Shree T, Sathe A, et al. Site to site comparison of follicular lymphoma biopsies by single cell RNA sequencing. American Society of Hematology meeting 2019, abstract #297. Orlando, December 7-10, 2019.

22. Andor N, Simonds EF, Czerwinski DK, et al. Single-cell RNA-Seq of follicular lymphoma reveals malignant B-cell types and coexpression of T-cell immune checkpoints. Blood 2019;133:1119–29.

23. Hude I, Sasse S, Engert A, et al. The emerging role of immune checkpoint inhibition in malignant lymphoma. Haematologica 2017;102:30–42.

24. Xu-Monette ZY, Zhou J, Young KH. PD-1 expression and clinical PD-1 blockade in B-cell lymphomas. Blood 2018;131:68–83.

25. Goodman A, Patel SP, Kurzrock R. PD-1-PD-L1 immune-checkpoint blockade in B-cell lymphomas. Nat Rev Clin Oncol 2017;14:203–20.

26. Andrews LP, Yano H, Vignali DAA. Inhibitory receptors and ligands beyond PD-1, PD-L1 and CTLA-4 : breakthroughs or backups. Nat Immunol 2019;20:1425–34.

27. Laurent C, Charmpi K, Gravelle P, et al. Several immune escape patterns in non-Hodgkin's lymphomas. Oncoimmunology 2015;4:e1026530.

28. Gribben JG, Fowler N, Morschhauser F. Mechanisms of action of lenalidomide in B-cell non-Hodgkin lymphoma. J Clin Oncol 2015;33:2803–11.

29. Vo DN, Alexia C, Allende-Vega N, et al. NK cell activation and recovery of NK cell subsets in lymphoma patients after obinutuzumab and lenalidomide treatment. Oncoimmunology 2017;7:e1409322.

30. Witzig TE, Wiernik PH, Moore T, et al. Lenalidomide oral monotherapy produces durable responses in relapsed or refractory indolent non-Hodgkin's lymphoma. J Clin Oncol 2009;27:5404–9.

31. Witzig TE, Vose JM, Zinzani PL, et al. An international phase II trial of single-agent lenalidomide for relapsed or refractory aggressive B-cell non-Hodgkin's lymphoma. Ann Oncol 2011;22:1622–7.

32. Chiu H, Trisal P, Bjorklund C, et al. Combination lenalidomide-rituximab immunotherapy activates anti-tumour immunity and induces tumour cell death by complementary mechanisms of action in follicular lymphoma. Br J Haematol 2019; 185:240–53.

33. Zucca E, Rondeau S, Vanazzi A, et al. Short regimen of rituximab plus lenalidomide in follicular lymphoma patients in need of first-line therapy. Blood 2019; 134:353–62.

34. Fowler NH, Davis RE, Rawal S, et al. Safety and activity of lenalidomide and rituximab in untreated indolent lymphoma: an open-label, phase 2 trial. Lancet Oncol 2014;15:1311–8.

35. Morschhauser F, Fowler NH, Feugier P, et al. Rituximab plus lenalidomide in advanced untreated follicular lymphoma. N Engl J Med 2018;379:934–47.

36. Leonard JP, Trneny M, Izutsu K, et al. AUGMENT: a phase III study of lenalidomide plus rituximab versus placebo plus rituximab in relapsed or refractory indolent lymphoma. J Clin Oncol 2019;37:1188–99.

37. Leonard JP, Jung SH, Johnson J, et al. Randomized trial of lenalidomide alone versus lenalidomide plus rituximab in patients with recurrent follicular lymphoma: CALGB 50401 (Alliance). J Clin Oncol 2015;33:3635–40.
38. Wang M, Fowler N, Wagner-Bartak N, et al. Oral lenalidomide with rituximab in relapsed or refractory diffuse large cell, follicular and transformed lymphoma: a phase II clinical trial. Leukemia 2013;27:1902–9.
39. Sharman J, Coleman M, Yacoub A, et al. Interim analysis of phase IIIB MAGNIFY study of induction R2 followed by maintenance in patients with relapsed/refractory indolent non-Hodgkin lymphoma. International Conference on Malignant Lymphoma 2019, abstract #70. Lugano, June 18-22, 2019 .
40. O'Nions J, Townsend W. The role of obinutuzumab in the management of follicular lymphoma. Future Oncol 2019;15:3565–78.
41. Klein C, Bacac M, Umana P, et al. Combination therapy with the type II anti-CD20 antibody obinutuzumab. Expert Opin Investig Drugs 2017;26:1145–62.
42. Decaup E, Jean C, Laurent C, et al. Anti-tumor activity of obinutuzumab and rituximab in a follicular lymphoma 3D model. Blood Cancer J 2013;3:e131.
43. Sehn LH, Goy A, Offner FC, et al. Randomized phase II trial comparing obinutuzumab (GA101) with rituximab in patients with relapsed CD20+ indolent B-cell non-Hodgkin lymphoma: final analysis of the GAUSS study. J Clin Oncol 2015; 33:3467–74.
44. Pott C, Sehn LH, Belada D, et al. MRD response in relapsed/refractory FL after obinutuzumab plus bendamustine or bendamustine alone in the GADOLIN trial. Leukemia 2020;34:522–32.
45. Marcus R, Davies A, Ando K, et al. Obinutuzumab for the first-line treatment of follicular lymphoma. N Engl J Med 2017;377:1331–44.
46. Morschhauser F, Le Gouill S, Feugier P, et al. Obinutuzumab combined with lenalidomide for relapsed or refractory follicular B-cell lymphoma (GALEN): a multicentre, single-arm, phase 2 study. Lancet Haematol 2019;6:e429–37.
47. Morschhauser F, Salles GA, Casanovas RO, et al. A phase II LYSA study of obinutuzumab combined with lenalidomide for advanced untreated follicular B-cell lymphoma in need of systemic therapy. Blood 2018;132(supplement 1):446.
48. Morschhauser F, Ghosh N, Lossos I, et al. Efficacy and safety of obinutuzumab + lenalidomide + atezolizumab in patients with relapsed or refractory follicular lymphoma: primary analysis of a phase 1b/2 trial. International Conference on Malignant Lymphoma 2019, abstract #68. Lugano, June 18-22, 2019.
49. Advani R, Flinn I, Popplewell L, et al. CD47 blockade by Hu5F9-G4 and rituximab in non-Hodgkin's lymphoma. N Engl J Med 2018;379:1711–21.
50. Advani R, Bartlett NL, Smith SM, et al. The first-in-class anti-CD47 antibody HU5F9-G4+Rituximab induces durable responses in relapsed/refractory DLBCL and indolent lymphoma: interim phase 1b/2 results. International Conference on Malignant Lymphoma 2019, abstract #51. Lugano, June 18-22, 2019.
51. Chen YP, Kim HJ, Wu H, et al. SIRPα expression delineates subsets of intratumoral monocyte/macrophages with different functional and prognostic impact in follicular lymphoma. Blood Cancer J 2019;9(10):84.
52. Fiorcari S, Martinelli S, Bulgarelli J, et al. Lenalidomide interferes with tumor-promoting properties of nurse-like cells in chronic lymphocytic leukemia. Haematologica 2015;100:253–62.
53. Chester C, Sanmamed MF, Wang J, et al. Immunotherapy targeting 4-1BB: mechanistic rationale, clinical results, and future strategies. Blood 2018;131:49–57.
54. Alfaro C, Echeveste JI, Rodriguez-Ruiz ME, et al. Functional expression of CD137 (4-1BB) on T helper follicular cells. Oncoimmunology 2015;4:e1054597.

55. Segal NH, Logan TF, Hodi FS, et al. Results from an integrated safety analysis of urelumab, an agonist anti-CD137 monoclonal antibody. Clin Cancer Res 2017;23: 1929–36.
56. Qi X, Li F, Wu Y, et al. Optimization of 4-1BB antibody for cancer immunotherapy by balancing agonistic strength with FcγR affinity. Nat Commun 2019;10:2141.
57. Otáhal P, Průková D, Král V, et al. Lenalidomide enhances antitumor functions of chimeric antigen receptor modified T cells. Oncoimmunology 2015;5:e1115940.
58. Labrijn AF, Janmaat ML, Reichert JM, et al. Bispecific antibodies: a mechanistic review of the pipeline. Nat Rev Drug Discov 2019;18:585–608.
59. Budde LE, Sehn LH, Assouline S, et al. Mosunetuzumab, a full-length bispecific CD20/CD3 antibody, displays clinical activity in relapsed/refractory B-cell non-Hodgkin lymphoma (NHL): interim safety and efficacy results from a phase 1 study. American Society of Hematology meeting 2018, abstract #399, San Diego, December 1-4, 2018.
60. Dickinson MJ, Morschhauser FM, Iacoboni G, et al. CD20-TCB (RG6026), a novel "2:1" format T-cell engaging bispecific antibody, induces complete remissions in relapsed/refractory B-cell non-Hodgkin's lymphoma. International Conference on Malignant Lymphoma 2019, abstract #53. Lugano, June 18-22, 2019.
61. Topp MS, Arnason J, Advani R, et al. Anti-CD20 x anti-CD3 bispecific antibody in patients with relapsed/refractory B-cell non-Hodgkin lymphoma. International Conference on Malignant Lymphoma 2019, abstract #52. Lugano, June 18-22, 2019.
62. Bacac M, Colombetti S, Herter S, et al. CD20-TCB with obinutuzumab pretreatment as next-generation treatment of hematologic malignancies. Clin Cancer Res 2018;24:4785–97.
63. Hatterer E, Barba L, Noraz N, et al. Co-engaging CD47 and CD19 with a bispecific antibody abrogates B-cell receptor/CD19 association leading to impaired B-cell proliferation. MAbs 2019;11:322–34.
64. Dheilly E, Moine V, Broyer L, et al. Selective blockade of the ubiquitous checkpoint receptor CD47 is enabled by dual-targeting bispecific antibodies. Mol Ther 2017;25:523–33.
65. Claus C, Ferrara C, Xu W, et al. Tumor-targeted 4-1BB agonists for combination with T cell bispecific antibodies as off-the-shelf therapy. Sci Transl Med 2019; 11(496) [pii:eaav5989].

Phosphatidylinositol-3-Kinase Inhibition in Follicular Lymphoma

Ryan C. Lynch, MD[a,b], Ajay K. Gopal, MD[a,b],*

KEYWORDS

- Follicular lymphoma • Targeted therapy • Autoimmune toxicity
- Combination therapy • PI3 kinase

KEY POINTS

- Phosphatidylinositol-3-kinase inhibition in follicular lymphoma has response rates of about 50% in relapsed/refractory patients for whom there are limited standard options.
- However, there are few durable responses owing to disease progression and high rates of discontinuation owing to adverse events (primarily autoimmune toxicity).
- Phosphatidylinositol-3-kinaseδ-specific or phosphatidylinositol-3-kinaseδ/γ-specific inhibition (idelalisib and duvelisib respectively) is associated with higher rates of late autoimmune toxicity owing to effects on regulatory T-cell subsets.
- Phosphatidylinositol-3-kinaseα and phosphatidylinositol-3-kinaseβ inhibition seen with copanlisib can lead to hyperglycemia and hypertension because these isoforms are more ubiquitously expressed.
- Futures studies are evaluating alternate dosing and combination strategies that may maintain and improve efficacy while improving the safety profile.

INTRODUCTION

Although chemoimmunotherapy (combining an anti-CD20 monoclonal antibody with chemotherapy) is the standard frontline treatment for symptomatic or high tumor burden follicular lymphoma (FL),[1–3] this strategy becomes less effective in the second-line setting or later.[4] A better understanding of the molecular mechanisms of lymphomagenesis has led to the development of drugs that specifically target these pathways. The phosphatidylinositol-3-kinase (PI3K) pathway is an important signaling pathway in B-cell lymphomas that is essential for proliferation and survival.[5] We describe the landscape of PI3K inhibitors that have been approved or are being tested for FL.

Research Funding: K24CA184039, Frank and Betty Vandermeer, Sonya and Tom Campion.
[a] Division of Medical Oncology, Department of Medicine, University of Washington, Seattle, WA, USA; [b] Clinical Research Division, Fred Hutchinson Cancer Research Center, 617 Eastlake Avenue East CE3-300, Seattle, WA 98109, USA
* Corresponding author. Clinical Research Division, Fred Hutchinson Cancer Research Center, 617 Eastlake Avenue East CE3-300, Seattle, WA, 98109.
E-mail address: agopal@uw.edu

PHOSPHATIDYLINOSITOL-3-KINASE BACKGROUND

Phosphatidylinositol is a membrane-bound lipid with a 6-carbon inositol head that contains multiple hydroxyl groups.[5] Isoforms of PI3K can be activated through upstream signaling, generating PIP_3, which activates downstream pathways.[6] PI3K isoforms are differentially expressed in various tissues, with PI3Kδ and PI3Kγ isoforms expressed exclusively in hematopoietic cells, and PI3Kα and PI3Kβ more widely expressed in both hematopoietic and nonhematopoietic cells.[6,7] Alterations in the PI3K pathway and the inhibitory phosphatase and tensin homolog pathway are common in B-cell lymphomas and PI3K inhibitors may abrogate tonic B-cell receptor signaling.[8,9] In addition, preclinical models have found that genetic inactivation of PI3Kδ leads to inactivation of regulatory T cells and subsequent inhibition of tumorigenesis.[5,10] A strong preclinical rationale and ability to select specific pharmacologic compounds have led to numerous clinical trials examining the activity of PI3K inhibitors in hematologic malignancies including FL.

A summary of agents approved by the US Food and Drug Administration (FDA) is presented in **Table 1**, and a selected list of trials and updated results is found in **Table 2**.

APPROVED AGENTS
Idelalisib

Idelalisib is an oral PI3Kδ inhibitor that is highly selective for the δ isoform compared with the α, β, and γ isoforms.[8] The high response rates in a phase I study of patients

---

Table 1
Summary of FDA-approved PI3K inhibitors and indications

FDA Approved Agent	Indication	Isoform Targeted	Notable Adverse Effects
Idelalisib[13]	Relapsed FL in patients who have received at least 2 prior systemic therapies.	δ	Anemia (any grade 35%, grade 3+ 3%) Thrombocytopenia (any grade 24%, grade 3+ 6%) Neutropenia (any grade 51%, grade 3+ 22%) Diarrhea (any grade 51%, grade 3+ 14%) Nausea (any grade 28%, grade 3+ 3%) Increased aspartate aminotransferase/ alanine aminotransferase (any grade 53%, grade 3+ 14%) Black box warning—fatal and/or severe: Diarrhea/colitis: 14%–20% Pneumonitis: 4% Infections: 21%–48% Intestinal perforation (rate not reported)

(continued on next page)

Table 1 (continued)			
FDA Approved Agent	**Indication**	**Isoform Targeted**	**Notable Adverse Effects**
Copanlisib[65]	Relapsed FL who have received at least 2 prior systemic therapies	Pan class	Anemia (any grade 78%, grade 3+ 4%) Thrombocytopenia (any grade 65%, grade 3+ 8%) Neutropenia (any grade 63%, grade 3+ 27%) Hyperglycemia (any grade 95%, grade 3+ 48%) Diarrhea (any grade 36%, grade 3+ 5%) Hypertension (any grade 35%, grade 3+ 27%) Pneumonia (any grade 21%, grade 3+ 14%)
Duvelisib[66]	Relapsed or refractory FL after at least 2 prior systemic therapies.	δ, γ	Anemia (any grade 20%, grade 3+ 11%) Thrombocytopenia (any grade 17%, grade 3+ 10%) Neutropenia (any grade 34%, grade 3+ 30%) Diarrhea/colitis (any grade 50%, grade 3+ 23%) Rash (any grade 31%, grade 3+ 9%) Nausea (any grade 24%, grade 3+ <1%) Increased aspartate aminotransferase/alanine aminotransferase (any grade 37%/40%, grade 3+ 6%/8%) Black box warning - fatal and/or severe: Infection: 31% Diarrhea/colitis 18% Cutaneous reactions: 5% Pneumonitis: 5%

with relapsed/refractory indolent non-Hodgkin lymphoma (NHL)[11] prompted a phase II study.

This pivotal study[12] was a single-arm, open-label, phase II study of patients who had received at least 2 prior therapies for the following histologies: grade 1 to 3A FL, marginal zone lymphoma (splenic, nodal, and extranodal), and lymphoplasmacytic lymphoma. Patients must have been refractory to both rituximab and an alkylating agent as defined by inability to achieve a complete response (CR) or partial response or progression of disease within 6 months of completion of either treatment in combination or administered separately. Based on the phase I data,[11] the dose selected was 150 mg 2 times per day.[13]

There were 125 patients accrued to the study, including 72 patients with FL.[14] Among patients with FL, the overall response rate (ORR) was 56%, which included

Table 2
Selected trials of PI3K inhibitors in FL

Indication	Agent	Combination	Phase	Number of FL Patients Treated	Median Age (Range)	ORR (CR) %	Median PFS (Months)	Median DOR (Months)	Grade 3 + AEs	Discontinuation Rate Due to AEs
Relapsed (Single Agent)	Idelalisib[a,14]	—	IIb	72	62 (33–84) Includes iNHL	56% (14%)	11 (Includes iNHL)	10.8	65%	25% (Includes iNHL)
	Duvelisib[a,25]	-	IIb	83	65 (30–90, Includes iNHL)	42% (1%)	9.5 (Includes iNHL)	10.0 (Includes iNHL)	88% (Includes iNHL)	31% (Includes iNHL)
	Copanlisib[a,29]	-	II	104	63 (25–82, includes iNHL)	59% (14%)	11.2 (included iNHL)	22.6 (includes iNHL)	68% (includes iNHL)	16%
	Umbralisib[34]	-	I	17	64 (51–72, includes all lymphoma histologies)	53% (12%)	16 mo (includes iNHL)	9.3	Not reported[c]	10% (Includes all lymphoma histologies)
	ME-401[38]	39/48 without rituximab	Ib	48	65 (38–81)	79% (26%) (single-agent)	Not reported	Not reported	Not reported	Not Reported
	Parsaclisib[40]	-	I/II	9	65 (30–88, Includes all lymphomas)	78% (22%)	Not reported	Not reported	40% with SAE (B-cell histologies)	25% (All B-cell histologies)
Relapsed (Combination Therapy)	Duvelisib[54]	Rituximab +/- Bendamustine	I	29 (B-cell NHL)	67 (40–83)	61% (13%)	10.7 mo (5.3 mo with bendamustine)	5.0 mo (6.2 mo with bendamustine)	87% (Includes CLL + B-cell NHL)	24% (Includes CLL + B-cell NHL)
	Umbralisib[36]	Ublituximab	I	19	64 (26–86 (all lymphoma histologies)	44% (22%)	Not reached	20.3	Not reported[d]	26%

Upfront	Duvelisib[62]	Rituximab or Obinutuzumab	II	55	58 (no range reported)	Rituximab: 87% (22%) Obinutuzumab: 91% (18%)	Not reported	Not reported	50%	14%

If results for the FL subset are not available, then the entire cohorts results will be listed with histologies noted.

Abbreviations: MZL, marginal zone lymphoma; PFS, progression-free survival; R/R, relapsed/refractory.

[a] FDA approved.

[b] Must have rituximab refractory disease.

[c] Eighty-five grade 3+ adverse events were seen in 90 total lymphoma patients treated of all histologies, although this may include patients who experienced more than 1 grade 3+ adverse event.

[d] Nineteen grade 3+ adverse events seen in 24 patients with iNHL, although this may include patient who experienced more than 1 grade 3+ adverse event.

a CR rate of 14%. The median time to response was 2.6 months (range, 1.6–11.0) with a median duration of response of 10.8 months (range, 0–26.9) and a median progression-free survival of 11.0 months (95% confidence interval, 8.0–14.0). On the basis of this study, idelalisib was approved by the FDA for patients with relapsed/refractory FL who have received at least 2 prior therapies.

Several retrospective studies have identified early relapse after primary treatment with chemoimmunotherapy as a poor prognostic factor associated with inferior overall survival.[15,16] A retrospective post hoc analysis was performed on the phase II study[17] and identified 46 patients who received first-line chemoimmunotherapy, 37 (80%) of whom had progression within 24 months of starting treatment. Among this high-risk population, the ORR was 57% (CR rate of 14%), which highlighted the activity of idelalisib in early relapse patients refractory to rituximab/alkylator.

Most patients experienced at least 1 grade 1 adverse event (99%), and most patients had at least 1 grade 3+ adverse event as well (65%).[14] Hematologic adverse events were common, including neutropenia (any grade 51%, grade 3+ 22%), anemia (any grade 35%, grade 3+ 3%), and thrombocytopenia (any grade 24%, grade 3+ 6%). Gastrointestinal adverse events were common, including diarrhea (any grade 51%, grade 3+ 14%), nausea (any grade 28%, grade 3+ 3%), and abdominal pain (any grade 14%, grade 3+ 3%). Other nonhematologic adverse events include rash (any grade 19%, grade 3+ 3%), pneumonia (any grade 11%, grade 3+ 7%), and increased aspartate aminotransferase/alanine aminotransferase (any grade 53%, grade 3+ 14%). Owing to this toxicity, treatment was interrupted in 44% of patients, and ultimately led to discontinuation in 25% of patients.

Postmarketing follow-up and additional studies including those in chronic lymphocytic leukemia (CLL)/small lymphocytic lymphoma have led to several black box warnings for idelalisib.[18–22] These include fatal and/or serious hepatotoxicity (16%–18%), diarrhea/colitis (14%–20%), pneumonitis (4%), infections (21%–48%), and intestinal perforation (rate not reported). Interestingly, the rates of grade 3+ diarrhea/colitis and transaminitis were higher in treatment-naïve patients compared with relapsed refractory patients, which supports the current hypothesis that these toxicities are mediated by an autoimmune reaction.[19,22,23] These data also highlight the immunomodulatory potential of this class of drugs.

Duvelisib

Duvelisib is another oral PI3K inhibitor that has activity on both the δ and γ isoforms.[24] A phase I study showed activity in B-cell NHL, particularly indolent lymphomas, so an open label phase II study[25] was designed to better evaluate the efficacy of duvelisib 25 mg 2 times per day for relapsed/refractory indolent NHL (iNHL). Similar to the idelalisib study, all patients must have been refractory to both rituximab (monotherapy or in combination) and either chemotherapy or radioimmunotherapy. Patients must have had at least 1 prior chemotherapy regimen that contained either an alkylating agent or nucleoside analog.

This study enrolled 129 patients, including 83 patients with FL. By central review the ORR was 42%, including 1% CR with a median time to response of 1.87 months. Although the median duration of response was not reported in the FL-only population, the proportion of all patients with iNHL who remained in response for at least 6 months was 43%.

In the overall iNHL population, 88% of patients had at least 1 grade 3+ adverse event, most commonly neutropenia (25%), diarrhea (15%), thrombocytopenia (12%), febrile neutropenia (9%), colitis (5%), pneumonia (5%), aspartate aminotransferase elevation (5%), and alanine aminotransferase elevation (3%).[25] Deaths attributable to study drug occurred in 4% of patients, including 2 patients with severe skin toxicity, 1 patient with pancolitis, 1 patient with a viral infection, and 1 patient with febrile neutropenia who died of sepsis. Severe toxicity seen in this study and others[24,26] have led to several black box warnings.[27] These include fatal and/or serious infections (31%), fatal and/or serious diarrhea/colitis (18%), fatal and/or serious cutaneous reactions (5%), and fatal and or serious pneumonitis (5%).

Copanlisib

In contrast with idelalisib and duvelisib, copanlisib is an IV pan-class PI3K inhibitor with inhibition of primarily the α (0.5 nmol/L) and δ (0.7 nmol/L) isoforms compared with the β (3.7 nmol/L) and γ (6.4 nmol/L) isoforms.[28] The first in human phase I study showed particular activity in FL, with 6 of 6 patients achieving an objective response, including 1 CR.[28]

The single-arm phase II study in patients with iNHL used a dosing schedule of copanlisib 60 mg IV on days 1, 8, and 15 of a 28-day cycle until intolerance or progression.[29] Patients must have received at least 2 prior therapies, but in contrast with these studies, there was no requirement for rituximab or alkylator refractoriness. For example, whereas all 142 patients of all iNHL histologies who enrolled on the study had received prior rituximab and alkylating chemotherapy, only 43% were refractory to both rituximab and alkylators. Among the 104 patients with FL, the ORR was 59%, including 14% CR. The median duration of response was 12.2 months (range, 0–22.6 months).

The toxicity profile of copanlisib differs from that of the more selective PI3Kδ or PI3Kδ/γ inhibitors idelalisib and duvelisib because the α isoform is more ubiquitously expressed.[6,29] The most common grade 3+ adverse events seen in the overall study population include hyperglycemia (41%), hypertension (24%), neutropenia (24%), pneumonia (16%), diarrhea/colitis 6%, thrombocytopenia (7%), and aspartate aminotransferase elevation (2%).[29] Of note, 16% of patients discontinued therapy owing to an adverse event attributable to copanlisib, including pneumonitis (4%), lung infection (3%), and hyperglycemia (2%). The low rate of discontinuation owing to off tumor effects is likely due the transient nature of the hyperglycemia and hypertension. Adverse events of interest included pneumonitis (any grade 8%, grade 3+ 1%) and colitis (any grade 1%, grade 3+ 1%). Of note, this study evaluated adverse events using CTCAE v4.03[30] and there was a revision in version 5.0[31] that changed how hyperglycemia is evaluated. For example, v4.03 grades hyperglycemia based on the glucose value, so for example, grade 3 hyperglycemia is greater than 250 to 500 mg/dL. In contrast, v5.0 grades hyperglycemia based on interventions required. Therefore, an abnormal glucose above baseline that does not require intervention would be grade 1. For patients requiring an intervention, initiation of an oral agent would be grade 2, and initiation insulin therapy would be grade 3. It is not clear how many patients with grade 3 hyperglycemia in this study would have been downgraded with the new classification.

CAN WE IMPROVE THE SAFETY OF PHOSPHATIDYLINOSITOL-3-KINASE INHIBITION?
Umbralisib

There are several agents that target the PI3K pathway in various stages of development that hope to improve upon the efficacy and safety of the currently approved agent. Umbralisib is a PI3Kδ-selective inhibitor, with little activity on the other isoforms.[32] Interestingly, it also inhibits casein kinase 1ε (CK1ε), whose signaling may mediate and augment autoimmune toxicities typically seen in this class.[33] The phase I study in relapse/refractory lymphomas gave a preview of the broad activity of this agent. Among 17 patients evaluable for response, the ORR was 53%, including a CR rate of 12%. In this limited subset, the median duration of response for patients with FL was 9.3 months.

Among the 90 patients across all lymphoma histologies evaluable for safety, all grade gastrointestinal adverse events were common,[34] but grade 3+ gastrointestinal and autoimmune adverse events were less common. These include diarrhea (all grade 43%, grade 3+ 3%), nausea (all grades 42%, grade 3+ 1%), vomiting (all grades 28%, grade 3+ 0%), and constipation (all grade 15%, grade 3+ 1%). Transaminitis was seen in only 7 patients (8%), of whom 2 subsequently discontinued treatment owing to this toxicity. Serious adverse events occurred in 8% of patients, including pneumonia (3%), lung infection (1%), febrile neutropenia (1%), and colitis (2%). Only 10% of patients discontinued treated owing to adverse events. The preliminary safety and efficacy of this agent has led to the development of several studies both as a single agent and in combination.[35,36]

REDUCED DOSING STRATEGIES: MAINTAINING EFFICACY WHILE IMPROVING SAFETY?
ME-401

ME-401 is another potent PI3Kδ selective inhibitor that is, being evaluated in relapsed/refractory B-cell malignancies. The initial phase I study evaluated continuous daily oral dosing at 60 mg, 120 mg, or 180 mg.[37,38] Although ORRs for this with or without rituximab were 78% and 79%, respectively, 10 of 29 (34%) of the first patients treated with continuous dosing experienced a grade 3+ immune-related adverse event. The hypothesis for this was that off-tumor, on-target inhibition of regulatory T cells were responsible for these events with prolonged exposure. An intermittent dosing strategy was devised based on the kinetics of regulatory T cells. Patients would be treated for 7 days to fully inhibit PI3Kδ, then wait 21 days before beginning a new cycle to allow for plasma drug clearance and recovery of regulatory T cells. Among the subsequent 19 patients treated with the intermittent dosing strategy, only 2 (11%) experienced a grade 3+ adverse event. This strategy is being further evaluated in a randomized phase II study that will allocate patients to continuous or intermittent dosing of ME-401.[39]

Parsaclisib

A similar approach has developed with parsaclisib (INCB50465). A promising phase I study in relapsed/refractory B-cell malignancies demonstrated that 7 of 9 (78%) of the first FL participants achieving an objective response, including 2 CR (22%).[40] However, this outcome was overshadowed by toxicity in the overall cohort (n = 52) that included 40% of patients experiencing a serious adverse event with 25% discontinuing therapy as a result. Serious adverse events requiring discontinuation included colitis (6%), diarrhea (6%), hypotension (6%), and pneumonitis (1%). The Citadel-203 study is a randomized phase II study that will examine the safety and efficacy of a maintenance dosing strategies in relapsed/refractory FL.[41] Patients will be assigned to receive continuous daily dosing versus 8 weeks of continuous dosing followed by weekly dosing.

Duvelisib

Although duvelisib qualified for FDA approval based on a phase II study, discontinuations owing to toxicity suggested a limited duration of benefit for this agent.[25] For this reason, the TEMPO study was devised to examine an alternate dosing schedule.[42] This randomized phase II, open-label, 2-arm study compares 2 intermittent dosing schedules. One group will receive 25 mg by mouth 2 times per day for 10 weeks followed by 25 mg 2 times per day 2 weeks on and 2 weeks off, whereas the other group will only receive the intermittent dosing schedule of 2 weeks on and 1 week off. The primary end point of this study will be the ORR, and a comparison of adverse events will be a secondary end point.

OTHER AGENTS IN DEVELOPMENT

There are numerous other agents that target the PI3K pathway that are in various stages of development, most of which have limited preliminary data available. Bupar-lisib (BKM120) is a pan class PI3K inhibitor that has been tested in a phase II study of B-cell malignancies.[43] Surprisingly, the response rates in patients with FL were lower than those seen in other similar phase I/II studies. Patients with FL had an ORR of 25% with a median progression-free survival of 9.3 months. Tenalisib is a PI3Kδ/γ inhibitor with activity in relapsed/refractory lymphoid malignancies[44] and a phase II study is ongoing to assess its efficacy in relapsed/refractory iNHL.[45]

Other PI3K inhibitors have been developed and studied in lymphomas with limited or no available data as a single agent or in combination with other agents. These include ACP-319,[46] KA2237,[47] GDC-0941,[48] GSK1059615,[49] XL147,[50] and ARQ-092.[51] Multitarget agents that include PI3K have also been designed, like PQR309[52] (PI3K + mammalian target of rapamycin) and CUDC-907[53] (PI3K + histone deacety-lase). It is not clear, however, if any of these drugs will be further developed for hema-tologic malignancies.

COMBINATIONS IN RELAPSED SETTING

Several studies are underway to evaluate the combination of a PI3K inhibitor with other targeted agents with or without chemotherapy for FL. Only 1 study so far has mature data that have been presented in a peer-reviewed or abstract form. This study assigned patients to receive either duvelisib with rituximab or the same combination with bendamustine.[54] In the chemotherapy arm, several dose combinations of duve-lisib (25 mg, 50 mg, and 75 mg 2 times per day continuously) and bendamustine (90 mg/m^2 or 70 mg/m^2 on days 1 and 2 of a 28-day cycle). Separating the efficacy and safety profile of duvelisib alone is challenging owing to the combination therapy. Further, the cohort is composed of several NHL histologies, which may decrease its generalizability and dilute the results. In addition, it is not clear how many patients had been previously refractory to rituximab-based therapies. Among 46 patients (27 NHL including 14 FL and 19 CLL), the most common adverse events were neutropenia (48%), fatigue (41%), and rash (41%).

There are also several studies with copanlisib that seek to demonstrate improved outcomes with combination therapies. An ongoing multicenter international phase III study is examining the impact of copanlisib on the effect of chemoimmunotherapy in relapsed iNHL.[55] Patients must have had at least 1 but no more than 3 prior lines of therapy. Participants must not have been refractory to their last rituximab containing regimen and may receive either rituximab plus CHOP or rituximab plus bendamustine depending on prior therapies. Patients will be randomized to receive copanlisib or pla-cebo in combination with chemoimmunotherapy. The primary end point is improve-ment in progression-free survival with copanlisib compared with placebo. A safety run-in was conducted and did not demonstrate any concerns with standard copanlisib dosing, and accrual of the phase III portion is ongoing.[55] A separate phase III study is being conducted in patients with relapsed iNHL who are not rituximab refractory with copanlisib + rituximab versus placebo and rituximab.[56]

Even PI3K inhibitors without an FDA label for any indication are attempting to improve on earlier phase I/II results with novel combinations. A phase I dose finding study is underway, combining parsaclisib with rituximab, rituximab and bendamustine, or ibrutinib.[57] A separate single-arm study is combining parsaclisib with obinutuzumab and bendamustine.[58] A 3-arm, nonrandomized, parallel assignment study for relapsed iNHL of ME-401 alone, with rituximab, or with the BTK inhibitor zanubrutinib is currently accruing patients.[59] Early phase I/Ib data for umbralisib as well as umbralisib in combination with the anti-CD20 monoclonal antibody ublituximab were promising and led to the design of a larger study in multiple NHL histologies, which showed an ORR of 44% and CR rate of 22% in 17 patients with FL with a median duration of response of 20.3 months.[36,60] An ongoing study will randomize patients with relapsed/refractory FL with at least 2 prior lines of therapy to umbralisib, ublituximab, or the combination of umbralisib and ublituximab.[61] In addition, a larger cooperative group study[35] was designed to improve outcomes in patients with FL with relapse within 2 years of primary chemoimmunotherapy, which in multiple retrospective studies have been shown to have inferior overall survival.[15,16] This study will randomize up to 150 patients to the combinations of umbralisib plus obinutuzumab, obinutuzumab and lenalidomide, or obinutuzumab with combination chemotherapy (CHOP or bendamustine depending on prior therapy).

STUDIES IN UPFRONT SETTING

Low-intensity chemotherapy-free approaches for the frontline management of FL are attractive for patients who might trade fixed-duration therapy with more toxicity for an indefinite therapy with fewer side effects. There has been reluctance, however, to use PI3K inhibitors in this setting owing to the excess toxicity seen in patients with CLL treated with upfront idealisib.[19] In this study, treatment-naïve patients with CLL received up to 8 months of idelalisib (the last 6 months in combination with rituximab). Among the first 24 patients, 13 (54%) developed grade 3+ transaminitis with a median time to toxicity of 28 days. High levels of proinflammatory cytokines (CCL3 and CCL4) were seen, and a lymphocytic infiltrate was seen on liver biopsies from 2 different patients.

The activity of duvelisib in untreated FL was examined in a 2-arm study with parallel assignment with patients allocated 1:1 to either duvelisib with rituximab or duvelisib with obinutuzumab.[62] These combinations were highly active with ORR of the rituximab (n = 23) and obinutuzumab (n = 22) combinations were 87% and 91%, respectively. Although the rates of grade 3+ transaminitis were lower than with idelalisib in untreated CLL (rituximab combination 21%, obinutuzumab combination 15%), 64% of patients had a toxicity that required dose hold or reduction while on treatment. Of these patients, 11% to 15% had a grade 3+ infection that included *Pneumocystis carinii* pneumonia, respiratory syncytial virus pneumonia, and pyelonephritis. The study was closed early by the decision of the sponsor with no further plans for development of duvelisib for untreated patients with FL.

Because upfront chemoimmunotherapy is highly effective in FL, the ideal PI3K inhibitor for use in this setting would have lower rates of hematologic toxicity and infections. A response adapted study for untreated FL with copanlisib and rituximab has been designed and recruitment is ongoing.[63] Patients will receive 6 months of the combination of copanlisib and rituximab followed by response assessment. Those in CR will not receive further therapy, whereas those in partial response will receive an additional 6 months of combination treatment. A phase II study of the combination of umbralisib and ublituximab for untreated FL and small lymphocytic lymphoma will administer up to 1 year of ublituximab and up to 2 years of umbralisib to responding patients.[64]

There are no current phase III studies in patients with untreated FL of PI3K inhibitors alone or in combination that are currently enrolling patients that have the potential to change current practice. Longer term safety and efficacy data from ongoing studies will be necessary to determine if this approach has the potential to replace standard chemoimmunotherapy.

SUMMARY

Currently approved agents (copanlisib, duvelisib, and idelalisib) are effective in the treatment of relapsed and refractory FL, although short-term and long-term toxicities as well as limited durations of response as a single agent warrant further investigations to improve the safety and efficacy of drugs in this class. Choosing among approved agents requires an analysis of patient comorbidities and treatment preferences. For example, 1 consideration is that copanlisib was not tested in a rituximab-refractory patient population, whereas idelalisib and duvelisib showed efficacy even in this high-risk population. Regardless of PI3K inhibitor selected, one should also consider that the prescriber information for idelalisib and duvelisib mandate *P carinii* pneumonia prophylaxis, while copanlisib recommends *P carinii* pneumonia prophylaxis be considered. It is also not clear how approved PI3K inhibitors should be sequenced with the recent FDA approval of lenalidomide plus rituximab, although one might expect PI3K inhibition to be used after this regimen based on the label (≥ 1 prior vs ≥ 2 prior lines of therapy). The study that led to the approval of lenalidomide used a rituximab combination in patients who were not refractory to CD20 antibodies, limiting cross-trial comparison. Except for the cooperative group early relapse FL study, there are unfortunately no current randomized studies comparing 2 different novel targeted agents that are approved for FL. Future directions in this field will examine the safety and efficacy of combination therapy as well as alternate dosing schedules that reduce toxicity may allow for patients to be treated on this class of drugs for longer periods of time. As always, enrollment ion clinical trials for patients with relapsed/refractory FL is strongly encouraged.

REFERENCES

1. Rummel MJ, Niederle N, Maschmeyer G, et al. Bendamustine plus rituximab versus CHOP plus rituximab as first-line treatment for patients with indolent and mantle-cell lymphomas: an open-label, multicentre, randomised, phase 3 non-inferiority trial. Lancet 2013;381:1203–10.

2. Flinn IW, van der Jagt R, Kahl BS, et al. Randomized trial of bendamustine-rituximab or R-CHOP/R-CVP in first-line treatment of indolent NHL or MCL: the BRIGHT study. Blood 2014;123:2944–52.

3. Marcus R, Davies A, Ando K, et al. Obinutuzumab for the first-line treatment of follicular lymphoma. N Engl J Med 2017;377:1331–44.

4. Sehn LH, Chua N, Mayer J, et al. Obinutuzumab plus bendamustine versus bendamustine monotherapy in patients with rituximab-refractory indolent non-Hodgkin lymphoma (GADOLIN): a randomised, controlled, open-label, multi-centre, phase 3 trial. Lancet Oncol 2016;17:1081–93.

5. Lampson BL, Brown JR. PI3Kdelta-selective and PI3Kalpha/delta-combinatorial inhibitors in clinical development for B-cell non-Hodgkin lymphoma. Expert Opin Investig Drugs 2017;26:1267–79.

6. Vanhaesebroeck B, Guillermet-Guibert J, Graupera M, et al. The emerging mechanisms of isoform-specific PI3K signalling. Nat Rev Mol Cell Biol 2010;11:329–41.

7. Clayton E, Bardi G, Bell SE, et al. A crucial role for the p110delta subunit of phosphatidylinositol 3-kinase in B cell development and activation. J Exp Med 2002; 196:753–63.

8. Lannutti BJ, Meadows SA, Herman SE, et al. CAL-101, a p110delta selective phosphatidylinositol-3-kinase inhibitor for the treatment of B-cell malignancies, inhibits PI3K signaling and cellular viability. Blood 2011;117:591–4.

9. Meadows SA, Vega F, Kashishian A, et al. PI3Kdelta inhibitor, GS-1101 (CAL-101), attenuates pathway signaling, induces apoptosis, and overcomes signals from the microenvironment in cellular models of Hodgkin lymphoma. Blood 2012;119:1897–900.

10. Ali K, Soond DR, Pineiro R, et al. Inactivation of PI(3)K p110delta breaks regulatory T-cell-mediated immune tolerance to cancer. Nature 2014;510:407–11.

11. Benson DM, Kahl BS, Furman RR, et al. Final results of a phase I study of idelalisib, a selective inhibitor of PI3Kδ, in patients with relapsed or refractory indolent non-Hodgkin lymphoma (iNHL). J Clin Oncol 2013;31:8526.

12. Gopal AK, Kahl BS, de Vos S, et al. PI3Kdelta inhibition by idelalisib in patients with relapsed indolent lymphoma. N Engl J Med 2014;370:1008–18.

13. Miller BW, Przepiorka D, de Claro RA, et al. FDA approval: idelalisib monotherapy for the treatment of patients with follicular lymphoma and small lymphocytic lymphoma. Clin Cancer Res 2015;21:1525–9.

14. Salles G, Schuster SJ, de Vos S, et al. Efficacy and safety of idelalisib in patients with relapsed, rituximab- and alkylating agent-refractory follicular lymphoma: a subgroup analysis of a phase 2 study. Haematologica 2017;102:e156–9.

15. Casulo C, Byrtek M, Dawson KL, et al. Early relapse of follicular lymphoma after rituximab plus cyclophosphamide, doxorubicin, vincristine, and prednisone defines patients at high risk for death: an analysis from the National LymphoCare Study. J Clin Oncol 2015;33:2516–22.

16. Maurer MJ, Bachy E, Ghesquieres H, et al. Early event status informs subsequent outcome in newly diagnosed follicular lymphoma. Am J Hematol 2016;91: 1096–101.

17. Gopal AK, Kahl BS, Flowers CR, et al. Idelalisib is effective in patients with high-risk follicular lymphoma and early relapse after initial chemoimmunotherapy. Blood 2017;129:3037–9.

18. Gilead Sciences Inc: Idelalisib prescriber information, Revised 10/2018, Available at: https://www.gilead.com/-/media/files/pdfs/medicines/oncology/zydelig/zydelig_pi.pdf. Accessed September 19, 2019,

19. Lampson BL, Kasar SN, Matos TR, et al. Idelalisib given front-line for treatment of chronic lymphocytic leukemia causes frequent immune-mediated hepatotoxicity. Blood 2016;128:195–203.

20. Brown JR, Byrd JC, Coutre SE, et al. Idelalisib, an inhibitor of phosphatidylinositol 3-kinase p110delta, for relapsed/refractory chronic lymphocytic leukemia. Blood 2014;123:3390–7.

21. Sharman JP, Coutre SE, Furman RR, et al. Final results of a randomized, phase III study of rituximab with or without idelalisib followed by open-label idelalisib in patients with relapsed chronic lymphocytic leukemia. J Clin Oncol 2019;37: 1391–402.

22. O'Brien SM, Lamanna N, Kipps TJ, et al. A phase 2 study of idelalisib plus rituximab in treatment-naive older patients with chronic lymphocytic leukemia. Blood 2015;126:2686–94.

23. Chellappa S, Kushekhar K, Munthe LA, et al. The PI3K p110delta isoform inhibitor idelalisib preferentially inhibits human regulatory T cell function. J Immunol 2019; 202:1397–405.
24. Flinn IW, O'Brien S, Kahl B, et al. Duvelisib, a novel oral dual inhibitor of PI3K-δ,γ, is clinically active in advanced hematologic malignancies. Blood 2018;131: 877–87.
25. Flinn IW, Miller CB, Ardeshna KM, et al. DYNAMO: a phase II study of Duvelisib (IPI-145) in patients with refractory indolent non-Hodgkin lymphoma. J Clin Oncol 2019;37:912–22.
26. Flinn IW, Hillmen P, Montillo M, et al. Results from the phase 3 DUO™ Trial: a randomized comparison of Duvelisib Vs Ofatumumab in patients with relapsed/refractory chronic lymphocytic leukemia or small lymphocytic lymphoma. Blood 2017;130:493.
27. Verastem Inc: Duvelisib prescriber information, Revised 9/2018. Available at: https://www.verastem.com/wp-content/uploads/2018/08/prescribing-information.pdf. Accessed September 20, 2019.
28. Patnaik A, Appleman LJ, Tolcher AW, et al. First-in-human phase I study of copanlisib (BAY 80-6946), an intravenous pan-class I phosphatidylinositol 3-kinase inhibitor, in patients with advanced solid tumors and non-Hodgkin's lymphomas. Ann Oncol 2016;27:1928–40.
29. Dreyling M, Santoro A, Mollica L, et al. Phosphatidylinositol 3-kinase inhibition by Copanlisib in relapsed or refractory indolent lymphoma. J Clin Oncol 2017; 35(35):3898–905.
30. Common Terminology Criteria for Adverse Events (CTCAE) v4.03. 2010. Available at: https://ctep.cancer.gov/protocolDevelopment/electronic_applications/docs/CTCAE_4.03.xlsx. Accessed September 20 2019.
31. Common Terminology Criteria for Adverse Events (CTCAE) v5.0. 2017. Available at: https://ctep.cancer.gov/protocolDevelopment/electronic_applications/ctc.htm#ctc_50. Accessed September 20, 2019.
32. Burris HA, Patel MR, Brander DM, et al. TGR-1202, a novel once daily PI3Kδ inhibitor, demonstrates clinical activity with a favorable safety profile, lacking hepatotoxicity, in patients with chronic lymphocytic leukemia and B-cell lymphoma. Blood 2014;124:1984.
33. Maharaj KK, Powers J, Fonseca R, et al. Abstract 545: differential regulation of human T-cells by TGR-1202, a novel PI3Kδ inhibitor. Cancer Res 2016;76:545.
34. Burris HA 3rd, Flinn IW, Patel MR, et al. Umbralisib, a novel PI3Kdelta and casein kinase-1epsilon inhibitor, in relapsed or refractory chronic lymphocytic leukaemia and lymphoma: an open-label, phase 1, dose-escalation, first-in-human study. Lancet Oncol 2018;19:486–96.
35. Obinutuzumab with or without Umbralisib, Lenalidomide, or combination chemotherapy in treating patients with relapsed or refractory grade I-IIIa follicular lymphoma. Available at: https://ClinicalTrials.gov/show/NCT03269669. Accessed September 23, 2019.
36. Lunning M, Vose J, Nastoupil L, et al. Ublituximab and Umbralisib in relapsed/refractory B-cell non-hodgkin lymphoma and chronic lymphocytic leukemia. Blood 2019;134(21):1811–20.
37. Soumerai JD, Pagel JM, Jagadeesh D, et al. Initial results of a dose escalation study of a selective and structurally differentiated PI3Kδ inhibitor, ME-401, in relapsed/refractory (R/R) follicular lymphoma (FL) and chronic lymphocytic leukemia (CLL)/small lymphocytic lymphoma (SLL). J Clin Oncol 2018;36:7519.

38. Zelenetz AD, Jagadeesh D, Reddy NM, et al. Results of the PI3Kδ inhibitor ME-401 alone or with rituximab in relapsed/refractory (R/R) follicular lymphoma (FL). J Clin Oncol 2019;37:7512.

39. Study of ME-401 in subjects with follicular lymphoma after failure of two or more prior systemic therapies. Available at: https://ClinicalTrials.gov/show/NCT03768505. Accessed September 23, 2019.

40. Ramchandren R, Phillips TJ, Wertheim M, et al. Ongoing phase 1/2 study of INCB050465 for relapsed/refractory (R/R) B-cell malignancies (CITADEL-101). J Clin Oncol 2017;35:7530.

41. An open-label study of INCB050465 in relapsed or refractory follicular lymphoma (CITADEL-203). Available at: https://ClinicalTrials.gov/show/NCT03126019. Accessed September 23, 2019.

42. A phase 2 study comparing 2 intermittent dosing schedules of Duvelisib in subjects with indolent non-hodgkin lymphoma. (TEMPO). Available at: https://ClinicalTrials.gov/show/NCT04038359. Accessed September 23, 2019.

43. Younes A, Salles G, Martinelli G, et al. Pan-phosphatidylinositol 3-kinase inhibition with buparlisib in patients with relapsed or refractory non-Hodgkin lymphoma. Haematologica 2017;102:2104–12.

44. Iyer SP, Huen A, Ferreri AJM, et al. Pooled safety analysis and efficacy of Tenalisib (RP6530), a PI3Kδ/γ inhibitor, in patients with relapsed/refractory lymphoid malignancies. Blood 2018;132:2925.

45. Efficacy and safety study of Tenalisib (RP6530), a Novel PI3K δ/γ dual inhibitor in patients with relapsed/refractory Indolent Non-Hodgkin's Lymphoma (iNHL). Available at: https://ClinicalTrials.gov/show/NCT03711578. Accessed September 23, 2019.

46. Acalabrutinib (ACP-196) in combination with ACP-319, for treatment of B-cell malignancies. Available at: https://ClinicalTrials.gov/show/NCT02328014. Accessed September 23, 2019.

47. The safety, pharmacokinetic and pharmacodynamic effect of KA2237 (PI3 Kinase p110β/δ Inhibitor) in B cell lymphoma. Available at: https://ClinicalTrials.gov/show/NCT02679196. Accessed September 23, 2019.

48. A study of GDC-0941 in patients with locally advanced or metastatic solid tumors or non-Hodgkin's lymphoma for which standard therapy either does not exist or has proven ineffective or intolerable. Available at: https://ClinicalTrials.gov/show/NCT00876122. Accessed September 23, 2019.

49. Phase I open-label, dose-escalation study of GSK1059615 in patients with solid tumors or lymphoma. Available at: https://ClinicalTrials.gov/show/NCT00695448. Accessed September 23, 2019.

50. Study of the safety and pharmacokinetics of XL147 (SAR245408) in adults with solid tumors or lymphoma. Available at: https://ClinicalTrials.gov/show/NCT00486135. Accessed September 23, 2019.

51. Phase 1 dose escalation study of ARQ 092 in adult subjects with advanced solid tumors and recurrent malignant lymphoma. Available at: https://ClinicalTrials.gov/show/NCT01473095. Accessed September 23, 2019.

52. Phase 2 study with PQR309 in relapsed or refractory lymphoma patients. Available at: https://ClinicalTrials.gov/show/NCT03127020. Accessed September 23, 2019.

53. Study to assess the safety, tolerability and pharmacokinetics of fimepinostat (CUDC-907) in patients with lymphoma. Available at: https://ClinicalTrials.gov/show/NCT01742988. Accessed September 23, 2019.

54. Flinn IW, Cherry MA, Maris MB, et al. Combination trial of Duvelisib (IPI-145) with rituximab or bendamustine/rituximab in patients with non-hodgkin lymphoma or chronic lymphocytic leukemia. Am J Hematol 2019;94(12):1325–34.
55. Gerecitano J, Santoro A, Leppä S, et al. Safety run-in of copanlisib in combination with rituximab plus bendamustine in patients with relapsed indolent non-hodgkin's lymphoma. Hematol Oncol 2017;35:408–10.
56. Copanlisib and Rituximab in Relapsed Indolent B-cell Non-Hodgkin's Lymphoma (iNHL). Available at: https://ClinicalTrials.gov/show/NCT02367040. Accessed September 23, 2019.
57. INCB050465 in combination with Rituximab, Bendamustine and Rituximab, or Ibrutinib in participants with previously treated B-Cell Lymphoma (CITADEL-112). Available at: https://ClinicalTrials.gov/show/NCT03424122. Accessed September 23, 2019.
58. Study evaluating safety and efficacy of INCB050465 combined with bendamustine and obinutuzumab in relapsed or refractory follicular lymphoma (CITADEL-102). Available at: https://ClinicalTrials.gov/show/NCT03039114. Accessed September 23, 2019.
59. A Study of ME-401 in Subjects With CLL/SLL, FL, and B-cell Non Hodgkin's Lymphoma. Available at: https://ClinicalTrials.gov/show/NCT02914938. Accessed September 23, 2019.
60. Burris HA, Flinn I, Lunning MA, et al. Long-term follow-up of the PI3Kδ inhibitor TGR-1202 to demonstrate a differentiated safety profile and high response rates in CLL and NHL: integrated-analysis of TGR-1202 monotherapy and combined with ublituximab. J Clin Oncol 2016;34:7512.
61. Study to assess the efficacy and safety of Ublituximab + TGR-1202 with or without Bendamustine and TGR-1202 alone in patients with previously treated Non-Hodgkins Lymphoma. Available at: https://ClinicalTrials.gov/show/NCT02793583. Accessed September 23, 2019.
62. Casulo C, Sancho J-M, Van Eygen K, et al. Contempo: preliminary results in first-line treatment of follicular lymphoma with the oral dual PI3K-δ,γ inhibitor, duvelisib, in combination with Rituximab or Obinutuzumab. Blood 2016;128:2979.
63. Response-adapted therapy with copanlisib and rituximab in untreated follicular lymphoma. Available at: https://ClinicalTrials.gov/show/NCT03789240. Accessed September 23, 2019.
64. Study to assess Umbralisib plus Ublituximab in patients with treatment naïve follicular lymphoma. Available at: https://ClinicalTrials.gov/show/NCT03828448. Accessed September 23, 2019.
65. Markham A. Copanlisib: first global approval. Drugs 2017;77:2057–62.
66. Blair HA. Duvelisib: first global approval. Drugs 2018;78:1847–53.

Novel Agents Beyond Immunomodulatory Agents and Phosphoinositide-3-Kinase for Follicular Lymphoma

Collin K. Chin, MBBS, Loretta J. Nastoupil, MD*

KEYWORDS

- Follicular lymphoma • POD24 • Novel agents • Checkpoint inhibitors
- BCL2 inhibitors • Epigenetic therapies • Bispecific antibodies
- Antibody-drug conjugates

KEY POINTS

- Understanding the molecular drivers of lymphomagenesis in follicular lymphoma and the role of the tumor microenvironment has led to the development of targeted novel therapies.
- Patients with relapsed/refractory follicular lymphoma who have progression of disease; fail allogeneic stem cell transplantation; harbor molecular markers suggesting chemoresistance; or progress after chimeric antigen receptor T-cell therapy are likely to benefit from novel agents.
- Combinations of novel agents have led to unprecedented outcomes in follicular lymphoma despite lackluster single-agent activity in the relapsed/refractory setting.
- Identification of patients with follicular lymphoma who are most likely to benefit from novel agents remains an area of need based on clinicopathologic and molecular features.

A POPULATION IN NEED

The standard treatment approach in most international centers for symptomatic, advanced stage follicular lymphoma (FL) is a combination of chemotherapy and monoclonal anti-CD20 antibody backbone.[1–3] The phase III RELEVANCE trial demonstrated similar efficacy between lenalidomide and rituximab (R2) as compared with rituximab, in combination with chemotherapy including cyclophosphamide, doxorubicin, vincristine, prednisone; bendamustine; or cyclophosphamide, vincristine, and prednisone with a more favorable safety profile potentially

Department of Lymphoma/Myeloma, University of Texas MD Anderson Cancer Center, 1515 Holcombe Boulevard, Unit 0429, Houston, TX 77030, USA
* Corresponding author.
E-mail address: lnastoupil@mdanderson.org

Hematol Oncol Clin N Am 34 (2020) 743–756
https://doi.org/10.1016/j.hoc.2020.03.002
0889-8588/20/© 2020 Elsevier Inc. All rights reserved.

adding to the long list of effective frontline treatment strategies.[4] However, 1 in 5 patients will have chemoresistant and/or refractory (R/R) disease or progression of disease within 24 months and have poor overall outcomes.[5] In patients with R/R disease, repeat biopsy is required to exclude disease transformation, which may be seen in up to 75% of patients with progression of disease within 24 months.[6] Patients who relapse with FL may proceed with high-dose salvage chemotherapy followed by either autologous or allogeneic stem cell transplantation (ASCT). In patients who are ineligible for ASCT or progress after ASCT, novel therapies as either as standard of care (immunomodulatory agents, BTK and phosphoinositide-3-kinase [PI3K] inhibitors) or on clinical trial are warranted. Despite our growing understanding of the molecular heterogeneity of FL, current treatment algorithms in FL are dogmatic and mandate a trial of chemotherapy as first or later lines of therapy. The M7-FLIPI was the first step in integrating our understanding of the molecular drivers of chemoresistant/refractory disease and identifies patients who may benefit from earlier and/or upfront treatment with novel agents.[7,8] There remains a need for new drug development to address the unmet need for patients with FL who have progression of disease within 24 months, progress after high-dose salvage chemotherapy and ASCT or are ineligible for ASCT, progress after BTK/PI3K failure, harbor molecular markers suggestive of R/R disease (M7-FLIPI), or have progressed after chimeric antigen receptor T-cell therapy.

MECHANISMS OF LYMPHOMAGENESIS AND THE TUMOR MICROENVIRONMENT

Traditional chemotherapy-based therapies exploit rapid cell division and various aspects of the cell cycle to induce apoptosis in neoplastic lymphoma cells. Although a blunt tool, chemotherapy has revolutionized the treatment of FL over the last half-century with the trade-off of significant off-target toxicities, including cytopenias, secondary infections, and chemotherapy-specific toxicity such as peripheral neuropathy and cardiotoxicity. Rituximab, the monoclonal anti-CD20 antibody, resulted in the single most significant improvement in overall survival in the last 2 decades.[9] Since then, our understanding of FL tumor biology has evolved, including the role of prosurvival mechanisms through B-cell receptor signaling pathways (BTK, PI3K, spleen tyrosine kinase [Syk]/Janus kinase, and cerebron signaling pathways), apoptosis pathways (BCL2 and BCL-xL), and epigenetic regulators (HDAC and EZH2). The tumor microenvironment and anergy of nonmalignant immune cells play a vital role in the development of FL with a demonstrable lack of tumor infiltrating T lymphocytes, expression of exhaustion markers on T lymphocytes and immune evasion by expression of inhibitory checkpoint markers including programmed cell death protein 1 (PD-1)/programmed cell death protein ligand-1 (PDL-1), LAG3, and CD47.[10–13]

Our growing understanding of the various components contributing to lymphomagenesis in FL have paved the way for novel therapies targeting specific pathways with promising activity in early phase clinical trials (**Fig. 1**). Additionally, novel antibody-based constructs and immune effector cell therapies have been developed to target specific surface antigens on FL cells including CD19, CD20, CD22, and CD79b. The current challenges now facing researchers are (1) describing and managing the unique and variable toxicity profiles of novel agents in addition to determining antilymphoma efficacy, (2) safely synergizing novel agents as doublet or triplet combinations with sound scientific rationale and avoiding unprecedented toxicity, (3) determining the optimal timing of therapy with novel agents (second line or later vs upfront) and (4) identifying the patient cohorts most likely to benefit based on clinicopathologic and molecular characteristics.

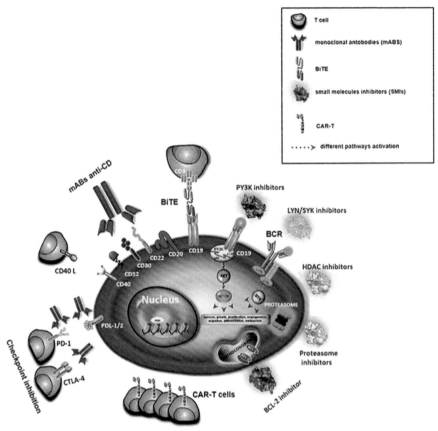

Fig. 1. Schematic diagram of the mechanism of action of novel agents in FL. (*From* Crisci S, Di Francia R, Mele S, Vitale P, Ronga G, De Filippi R, et al. Overview of Targeted Drugs for Mature B-Cell Non-hodgkin Lymphomas. Front Oncol. 2019;9:443; https://doi.org/10.3389/fonc.2019.00443.)

NOVEL THERAPIES

In this review, we describe the current evidence for novel therapies available for FL in the R/R and upfront settings (**Table 1**). The role of immunomodulatory agents, BTK inhibitors, P13K inhibitors, and chimeric antigen receptor T-cell therapy are described in separate articles.

IMMUNE CHECKPOINT INHIBITORS

Immune checkpoints are vital in facilitating immune and tumor cell interactions and effector mechanisms within the tumor microenvironment. Neoplastic lymphoma cells escape immune surveillance by expressing ligands including PDL-1, lymphocyte activation gene 3, and CD47 to evade detection by T lymphocytes and macrophages.

The PD-1 axis represents the first immune checkpoint to be investigated within non-Hodgkin lymphomas (NHLs) and exists to regulate immune responses of activated T cells to infection and prevent autoimmunity.[14,15] PD-1 binding to its ligands PDL-1 and PDL-2 sends inhibitory signals, which leads to activated T-cell apoptosis.[16]

Table 1
Summary of investigational novel agents in the treatment of FL

Novel Agent Class and Name	Phase	Design	Population (n)	Outcomes
Immune checkpoint inhibitors				
Pembrolizumab	II[18]	Single arm study in combination with rituximab	R/R FL (n = 27)	ORR 80%, CR 60%, median FU 7 mo
Nivolumab	II[19]	Single arm study in combination with rituximab	Front line FL (n = 19)	ORR 84%, CR 47%, median FU 17 mo
Atezolizumab	I/IIb[69]	Single arm study in combination with lenalidomide and obinutuzumab	R/R FL (n = 38)	CR 72%
Hu5F9-G4	I/IIb[25]	Single arm study in combination with rituximab	R/R B-cell NHL (FL n = 7)	ORR 71%, CR 43%, median FU 8.1 mo
Epigenetic transcriptional modifiers				
Tazemetostat	II[41]	Single arm study of single agent tazemetostat	R/R FL; EZH2 mutated and WT (n = 99)	EZH2 MT—ORR 77%, CR 7%, median PFS 11.1 mo
Abexinostat	II[37]	Single arm study of single agent abexinostat	R/R NHL or chronic lymphocytic leukemia (FL n = 14)	EZH WT—ORR 34%, CR 6%, median PFS 5.7 mo FL—ORR 56% Median PFS 20.5 mo
Vorinostat	II[32]	Single arm study of single agent vorinostat	R/R FL (n = 17)	ORR 47%, CR 24% Median PFS 15.6 mo
BCL-2 inhibitors				
Venetoclax	I[45] II[70]	Single arm study of single agent venetoclax In combination with rituximab and/or bendamustine	R/R B-cell NHL (FL n = 29) R/R FL (n = 164)	ORR 38%, CR 14% Median PFS 11 mo Ven + R = ORR 33% Ven + BR = ORR 68%

B-cell receptor pathway inhibitors				
Cerdulatinib	II[53]	Single agent or in combination with rituximab	R/R FL (n = 59)	C = ORR 45% (CR 12.5%) C + R = ORR 60% (CR 12%)
Antibody–drug conjugates				
Polatuzumab vedotin	II[56]	Pinatuzumab vedotin or polatuzumab vedotin in combination with either rituximab or obinutuzumab	R/R FL (n = 230)	ORR 70%, CR 45%
	II[57]	In combination with bendamustine and rituximab	R/R FL (n = 45)	ORR 76%, CR 44% (2.4 mg/kg) Median PFS 15 mo
	II[59]	In combination with lenalidomide and obinutuzumab	R/R FL (n = 56)	ORR 76% CR 65% Median PFS not reached, median FU 11.3 mo
Radioimmunotherapy				
Ibritumomab tiuxetan	III[63]	Randomized controlled trial of Ibritumomab tiuxetan vs rituximab monotherapy	R/R low-grade B-cell NHL (FL n = 137)	*Untreated FL* = ORR 100% CR 93%, median PFS 4.1 y *R/R FL* = ORR 93%, CR 73%, median PFS 2.2 y
Bispecific antibodies				
Mosunetuzumab	I/Ib[71]	Single arm study with single agent	R/R B-cell NHL (FL n = 69)	ORR 53%, CR 31%
RG6026 (CD20-TCB)	I/Ib[72]	Single arm study with single agent	R/R B-cell NHL (FL n = 8)	ORR 63%, CR 50%
	I/Ib[67]	Single arm study in combination with obinutuzumab	R/R B-cell NHL (FL n = 5)	ORR 80% CR 80% (100% CR rate at 16 mg dose level)

Abbreviations: BR, bendamustine and rituximab; FU, follow-up.

PD-1 is also present on regulatory T cells, natural killer cells, B cells, and therefore PD-1 blockage results in (1) enhancement antitumor cytotoxicity by downregulation of regulatory T cells and increased natural killer cell killing, and (2) reactivation of exhausted T cells.[17] Pembrolizumab, an anti–PD-1 monoclonal antibody, has been investigated in a phase II trial in combination with rituximab in R/R FL with an overall response rate (ORR) of 80% and complete response (CR) rate of 60%, although follow-up was limited, at a median of 7 months.[18] Nivolumab, another anti-PD-1 monoclonal antibody has been investigated in a phase Ib/II trial in combination with rituximab in front-line treatment of FL with similar results with an ORR of 84%, a CR of 47%, and a median follow-up of 17 months.[19] Toxicity profiles of PD-1 inhibitors has been as expected in the setting of FL, including rash, diarrhea, and pneumonitis. However, the true activity of PD-1 inhibition is somewhat debatable with the lack of phase III trials where the published data of rituximab monotherapy have shown similar response rates with an ORR of 75% and CR 38%.[20] This finding has been supported by recent preclinical studies demonstrating that dual checkpoint blockade may be required to overcome the T-cell exhaustion phenotype, with clinical trials combining PD-1 inhibitors with lymphocyte activation gene 3 inhibitors now recruiting in R/R FL.[21]

CD47 is an antiphagocytic signal expressed by lymphoma cells to enable immune evasion of macrophages and other phagocytes.[22] Anti-CD47 antibodies can induce phagocytosis of tumor cells by blocking CD47 and its ligand signal regulatory protein alpha, as well as inducing a T-cell response by cross-presenting tumor antigens by phagocytes to T cells.[23,24] Hu5F9-G4 is a humanized CD47-blocking monoclonal antibody shown to have unprecedented activity in a phase Ib trial in combination with rituximab. In patients with R/R FL, the ORR was 71% and the CR was 43%, with 91% of responses ongoing at a median follow-up of 8 months.[25] Unlike other checkpoint inhibitors, Hu5F9-G4 selectively eliminates malignant cells by unmasking prophagocytic signals not expressed on normal cells with the exception of aging red cells.[26] As expected, the toxicity profile is minimal with the exception of transient anemia. Combination and frontline studies are planned.

Epigenetic Therapies

Translational studies in FL have demonstrated that deregulation of the epigenome is an initiating event with more than 95% of cases harboring at least 1 mutation in an epigenetic regulator.[7,27] In human malignancies, epigenetic silencing is characterized by histone deacetylation.[28,29] Histone deacetylase (HDAC) and histone acetyl transferases are enzymes that regulate deacetylation and acetylation of histone and nonhistone proteins, and therefore governing gene transcription, protein production, and cellular function.[30] HDAC inhibitors cause hyperacetylation of histones and activate genes involved in tumor suppression, cell growth, and apoptosis.[31] Potential dose-limiting toxicities include fatigue, thrombocytopenia, and QTc prolongation. Vorinostat is an oral HDAC inhibitor that has been investigated as monotherapy in phase II studies in R/R FL resulting in an ORR of 47% to 49% with a median progression-free survival (PFS) of 15.6 and 20.0 months.[32,33] The addition of rituximab did not improve overall response or durability of disease control, although a randomized comparison has not been performed.[34] Abexinostat is another oral HDAC inhibitor that is dosed twice daily to allow continuous exposure at therapeutic concentrations while avoiding high peak concentrations, which cause toxicity.[35] A phase II study of abexinostat in R/R NHL or chronic lymphocytic leukemia demonstrated an ORR of 28%; among patients with R/R FL, the ORR was 56% with a median PFS of 10.2 months.[36] Similar findings were found in a separate phase II study of abexinostat in R/R NHL, which showed an ORR of 56.3% at a median PFS of 20.5 months.[37] The toxicity profile was as expected with HDAC inhibitors, including nausea, diarrhea, and fatigue. Several other HDAC inhibitors are also being investigated in FL to address the loss of histone acetylation associated with CREBBP and EP300 mutations (panobinostat and mocetinostat).[38]

EZH2 is a gain-of-function mutation that results in increased H3K27 histone methylation and occurs in 25% of cases of FL.[39] This results in enhanced accumulation of hyperproliferative B lymphocytes after antigen exposure, repression of the tumor suppressor gene CDKN1A, low IRF4 levels, increased vascular endothelial growth factor expression, increased nuclear factor κB and RAS signaling, and improved cell survival.[30] Tazemetostat is an orally available small molecule inhibitor of EZH2 that has preclinical activity in EZH2 mutated and wild-type lymphomas.[40] A recent update of the large phase II trial investigating tazemetostat in R/R FL has shown higher response rates in EZH2 MT (ORR, 70%; CR, 7%; partial response, 70%) at a median PFS of 11.1 months (median duration of response, 8.3 months). In comparison, EZH2 WT have fewer responses (ORR, 34%; CR, 6%; partial response, 28%) at a median PFS of 5.7 months (median duration of response, 13.0 months).[41] Tazemetostat was very tolerable with few side effects, making it an attractive option for combination therapies.

BCL-2 INHIBITORS

Bcl-2 family proteins are key regulators of apoptosis in neoplastic cells and comprise of antiapoptotic proteins (Bcl-2 and Bcl-xL) and proapoptotic proteins (Bak, Bad, Bax, Noxa, and Puma).[42] The interaction of BH3-only proteins with Bax and Bak result in activation, mitochondrial permeabilization, and apoptosis.[43] BH-3 mimetics are a group of small molecules designed to bind to these proteins and promote apoptosis. Venetoclax (ABT-199) is an oral small molecule BH3-mimetic engineered to avoid Bcl-xL inhibition and off-target dose-limiting thrombocytopenia, a significant limitation with earlier BH-3 mimetics including ABT-737 and its derivative ABT-263 (navitoclax).[44] In a phase I study in R/R B-cell NHL, single-agent venetoclax had an ORR of 38% in FL (14% CR) and grade 3 or greater thrombocytopenia in 7% of patients.[45] However, in comparison with the superior activity in chronic lymphocytic leukemia and mantle cell lymphoma, the activity of venetoclax in FL was somewhat disappointing given the critical role Bcl-2 plays in the pathophysiology of FL. Recent studies have demonstrated that t(14;18) B cells are found in the blood of healthy individuals, which, although not directly causing FL, has been shown to increase the lifetime risk of developing FL.[46,47] Therefore, the acquisition of additional mutations are required for neoplastic transformation, suggesting that the pathogenesis of FL is more complex than a simplistic BCL2 gene translocation and BCL2 inhibition. Venetoclax has been shown to be synergistic with other novel agents including EZH2 inhibitors in-vitro, but are highly dependent on tumor expression of BCL2 translocations and EZH2 mutations.[48] A phase Ib study of venetoclax in combination with bendamustine and rituximab demonstrated an improved ORR in patients with R/R FL of 87% with apparent synergy and tolerability.[49] Multiple studies of venetoclax in combination therapy with chemotherapy and other novel therapies are underway in the R/R and frontline settings (NCT03980171, NCT02956382, and NCT02877550).

SPLEEN TYROSINE KINASE AND JANUS KINASE INHIBITORS

B-cell receptor kinase inhibitors, including BTK and PI3K inhibitors, are highly effective in the treatment of R/R FL but are ultimately not curative. Syk is a key regulator of B-cell receptor signaling upstream of BTK and PI3K.[50] Syk inhibitor single-agent therapy with entospletinib has demonstrated early clinical activity in patients with R/R FL, particularly after BTK and PI3K failure.[51] Additionally, FL has been shown to have greater number of follicular helper T cells that express high levels of IL-4, which support tumor growth and proliferation through the JAK and signal transducer and activator of transcription proteins signaling pathway via JAK1 and JAK3.[52] Cerdulatinib (PRT062070) is a dual JAK/Syk inhibitor which simultaneously inhibits both Syk and JAK1/3 and has demonstrated activity in R/R FL in a phase II study.[53] As a single agent, the ORR was 45% (12.5% CR) with marginally improved outcomes when combined with rituximab (ORR, 60%; CR ,12%). Durable responses were seen with the most common grade 3 or higher adverse events being raised lipase (27%), neutropenia (18%), infection (18%), and diarrhea (12%). The study is still recruiting in the combination cohort (NCT01994382).

ANTIBODY–DRUG CONJUGATES

Antibody–drug conjugates are anticancer agents linked to monoclonal antibodies with varied success in R/R FL. Inotuzumab ozagamicin, which is composed of an anti-CD22 monoclonal antibody with calicheamicin, was terminated in a phase III study in R/R aggressive NHL owing to futility.[54,55] Polatuzumab vedotin (PoV) is an anti-CD79b monoclonal antibody conjugated to monomethyl aurostatin E, a microtubule toxin. In a phase II study of PoV monotherapy in R/R FL, the ORR was 70% and CR rate was 45%.[56] The most common grade 3 and greater toxicities were neutropenia and diarrhea. In a separate study of PoV in R/R FL the ORR and CR rates were 76% and 44%, respectively, at the higher dose level of 2.4 mg/kg, although higher rates of discontinuation were noted compared with the lower dose cohort owing to grade 2 to 4 peripheral neuropathy (72% vs 40%).[57] When combined with bendamustine and rituximab, PoV was not significantly better than bendamustine and rituximab alone in the treatment of R/R FL.[58] Similarly, PoV in combination with obinutuzumab/lenalidomide did not seem to significantly improve outcomes in R/R FL, although a randomized study has not been performed.[59,60] Ongoing studies of PoV in combination with alternative anti-CD20 monoclonal antibodies and/or chemotherapy are currently recruiting (NCT02600897 and NCT02611323).

RADIOIMMUNOTHERAPY

Radioimmunotherapy (RIT) regimens where radioisotopes are conjugated to antibodies (typically anti-CD20 antibodies) have been used to treat R/R FL. Prospective trials of RIT have demonstrated ORR of up to 80% in R/R FL.[61,62] Ibritumomab tiuxetan, a murine anti-CD20 monoclonal antibody conjugated to the radioisotope yttrium-90, has had a recent update of long-term outcomes with a median follow-up of 10.2 years.[63] In untreated FL, the ORR was 100% and the CR rate was 93%, and in R/R FL the ORR was 93% and the CR was 73%. The median PFS for the untreated cohort was 4.1 years versus 2.2 years in the R/R cohort. However, the main toxicities associated with RIT included grade 3 neutropenia (46%) and grade 3 thrombocytopenia (47%), which persisted up to 9 weeks after cessation of therapy.[61] Therefore, RIT provides a less toxic therapy for a select group of patients with few side effects, the most notable being cytopenias. However, the complexities associated with delivering this treatment and the availability of many other agents have limited its widespread uptake.

BISPECIFIC ANTIBODIES

Bispecific antibodies are immunoglobulin molecules containing 2 different antigen binding sites—one directed against the CD3 receptor activating cytotoxic T lymphocytes and the other against specific antigens of tumor cells.[64] The convergence and subsequent interaction of cytotoxic T lymphocytes and tumor cells owing to bispecific antibody binding activates cytotoxic T cells and destruction of tumor cells. Although first described in a therapeutic context in 1992, the first publication demonstrating activity of bispecific antibodies in R/R B-NHL was in 2008 with blinatumomab, a bispecific T-cell engager CD3/CD19 antibody.[65] The toxicity profile is similar to that of chimeric antigen receptor T cells with cytokine release syndrome and neurotoxicity occurring owing to rapid T-cell expansion and proliferation.

Mosunetuzumab (RG7828) is a full-length, fully humanized IgG1 bispecific antibody targeting CD3 and CD20. An ongoing phase I/Ib study has demonstrated ongoing efficacy and tolerability in patients with R/R indolent NHL (96% FL) with an ORR of 64% and a CR rate of 42%, with durability in responses with 93% of patients remaining in CR (median time from first CR of 5.8 months).[66] Seven percent of patients (5/72) had prior chimeric antigen receptor T-cell failure, indicating activity in this difficult-to-treat population. Cytokine release syndrome was seen in 28% of patients (mainly grade 1 or 2) mostly occurring in cycle one. Immune effector cell-associated neurotoxicity syndrome was rare and occurred in less than 2% of patients during cycles 1 and 2. Frequency of CRS and neurologic adverse events did not correlate to mosunetuzumab dose.

CD20-TCB (RG6026) is another novel T-cell engaging bispecific antibody with a unique 2:1 molecular format comprising 2 fragment antigen-binding regions that bind CD20 and CD3. The molecular format of CD20-TCB is thought to increase tumor antigen avidity, rapid T-cell activation, and enhanced tumor cell killing compared with other bispecific formats and the ability to combine with other CD20-targeted agents. In a phase I/Ib trial of CD20-TCB and obinutuzumab in patients with R/R B-cell NHL, the ORR and CR rate in FL was 80% (4 of 5 patients) with all patients (3 of 3) in CR at the maximum (16 mg) dose cohort.[67] cytokine release syndrome occurred in 57% of patients (mostly grade 1 or 2) with rare reports of neurotoxicity (21% grade 1 or 2, 4% grade 3). Newer bispecific antibody constructs are being investigated including IgM-based constructs with 10 binding sites and increased avidity and potency with lower risk of cytokine release syndrome and immune effector cell-associated neurotoxicity syndrome.[68]

SUMMARY

As our understanding of the pathogenesis of FL grows, the number of novel therapies targeting various signaling pathways, tumor microenvironment, and surface proteins have rapidly increased in the last decade. As numerous early phase clinical trials examining novel agents as single or combination therapies continue to recruit and mature, we are reminded that careful trial design is required to avoid unexpected toxicities and ensure efficacy. A range of novel therapies are highly active in the difficult-to-treat population of R/R FL, particularly those in need including post BTK/PI3K inhibitor failure, post-ASCT relapse, and post–chimeric antigen receptor T-cell failure, with several agents likely to receive approval from the US Food and Drug Administration in the near future. Additionally, the incorporation of novel therapies in the second or frontline settings are currently under investigation, which may yield improved outcomes as compared with the R/R setting. A significant deficiency still exists in identifying the patients most likely to benefit from specific novel agents based on clinicopathologic and molecular characteristics. Ongoing recruitment onto clinical trials is needed to further develop the area of novel therapies with significant changes in the treatment paradigm of relapsed or refractory FL expected within the next few years.

REFERENCES

1. National Cancer Institute. Surveillance, epidemiology, and end results (SEER) program. National Cancer Institute, Cold Spring Harbor: Harborside Press LLC, DCCPS; 2014.
2. El-Galaly TC, Bilgrau AE, de Nully Brown P, et al. A population-based study of prognosis in advanced stage follicular lymphoma managed by watch and wait. Br J Haematol 2015;169:435–44.
3. Junlen HR, Peterson S, Kimby E, et al. Follicular lymphoma in Sweden: nationwide improved survival in the rituximab era, particularly in elderly women: a Swedish Lymphoma Registry study. Leukemia 2015;29:668–76.
4. Morschhauser F, Fowler NH, Feugier P, et al. Rituximab plus lenalidomide in advanced untreated follicular lymphoma. N Engl J Med 2018;379:934–47.
5. Casulo C, Byrtek M, Dawson KL, et al. Early relapse of follicular lymphoma after rituximab plus cyclophosphamide, doxorubicin, vincristine, and prednisone defines patients at high risk for death: an analysis from the national lymphocare study. J Clin Oncol 2015;33:2516–22.
6. Sarkozy C, Trneny M, Xerri L, et al. Risk factors and outcomes for patients with follicular lymphoma who had histologic transformation after response to first-line immunochemotherapy in the PRIMA trial. J Clin Oncol 2016;34:2575–82.
7. Pastore A, Jurinovic V, Kridel R, et al. Integration of gene mutations in risk prognostication for patients receiving first-line immunochemotherapy for follicular lymphoma: a retrospective analysis of a prospective clinical trial and validation in a population-based registry. Lancet Oncol 2015;16:1111–22.
8. Li X, Kositsky R, Reddy A, et al: Whole Exome and Transcriptome Sequencing in 1042 Cases Reveals Distinct Clinically Relevant Genetic Subgroups of Follicular Lymphoma. Blood 2019;134(Supplement_1):19.
9. Colombat P, Salles G, Brousse N, et al. Rituximab (anti-CD20 monoclonal antibody) as single first-line therapy for patients with follicular lymphoma with a low tumor burden: clinical and molecular evaluation. Blood 2001;97:101–6.
10. Vallee A, Shourian M, Johnson N, et al. Evaluation of T-Cell Compartment By Complex Multiparameter Flow Cytometry Reveals Distinct Patterns of T-Cell Exhaustion in DLBCL, FL and HL Patients. Blood 2019;134(Supplement_1):2806.
11. Haebe S, Shree T, Sathe A, et al. Site to Site Comparison of Follicular Lymphoma Biopsies By Single Cell RNA Sequencing. Blood 2019;134(Supplement_1):297.
12. Nath K, Law SC, Sabdia MB, et al. Intra-Tumoral CD8+ T-Cells in Follicular Lymphoma Contain Large Clonal Expansions That Are Amenable to Dual-Checkpoint Blockade. Blood 2019;134(Supplement_1):2793.
13. Mondello P, Fama A, Larson M, et al. Intrafollicular CD4+ T-Cells As an Independent Predictor of Early Clinical Failure in Newly Diagnosed Follicular Lymphoma. Blood 2019;134(Supplement_1):121.
14. Freeman GJ, Long AJ, Iwai Y, et al. Engagement of the PD-1 immunoinhibitory receptor by a novel B7 family member leads to negative regulation of lymphocyte activation. J Exp Med 2000;192:1027–34.
15. Nishimura H, Nose M, Hiai H, et al. Development of lupus-like autoimmune diseases by disruption of the PD-1 gene encoding an ITIM motif-carrying immunoreceptor. Immunity 1999;11:141–51.
16. Francisco LM, Salinas VH, Brown KE, et al. PD-L1 regulates the development, maintenance, and function of induced regulatory T cells. J Exp Med 2009;206:3015–29.

17. Terme M, Ullrich E, Aymeric L, et al. IL-18 induces PD-1-dependent immunosuppression in cancer. Cancer Res 2011;71:5393–9.
18. Nastoupil LJ, Westin JR, Fowler NH, et al. Response rates with pembrolizumab in combination with rituximab in patients with relapsed follicular lymphoma: interim results of an on open-label, phase II study. J Clin Oncol 2017;35:7519.
19. Barraclough A, Chong G, Gilbertson M, et al. Immune Priming with Single-Agent Nivolumab Followed By Combined Nivolumab & Rituximab Is Safe and Efficacious for First-Line Treatment of Follicular Lymphoma; Interim Analysis of the '1st FLOR' Study. Blood 2019;134 (Supplement_1):1523.
20. Martinelli G, Schmitz SF, Utiger U, et al. Long-term follow-up of patients with follicular lymphoma receiving single-agent rituximab at two different schedules in trial SAKK 35/98. J Clin Oncol 2010;28:4480–4.
21. Armand P, Zinzani PL, Palcza J, et al. Phase 1-2 Study of Pembrolizumab Combined with the Anti–LAG-3 Antibody MK-4280 for the Treatment of Hematologic Malignancies. Blood 2019;134(Supplement_1):1548.
22. Jaiswal S, Jamieson CH, Pang WW, et al. CD47 is upregulated on circulating hematopoietic stem cells and leukemia cells to avoid phagocytosis. Cell 2009;138:271–85.
23. Chao MP, Alizadeh AA, Tang C, et al. Anti-CD47 antibody synergizes with rituximab to promote phagocytosis and eradicate non-Hodgkin lymphoma. Cell 2010;142:699–713.
24. Tseng D, Volkmer JP, Willingham SB, et al. Anti-CD47 antibody-mediated phagocytosis of cancer by macrophages primes an effective antitumor T-cell response. Proc Natl Acad Sci U S A 2013;110:11103–8.
25. Advani R, Flinn I, Popplewell L, et al. CD47 blockade by Hu5F9-G4 and rituximab in non-Hodgkin's lymphoma. N Engl J Med 2018;379:1711–21.
26. Liu J, Wang L, Zhao F, et al. Pre-clinical development of a humanized anti-CD47 antibody with anti-cancer therapeutic potential. PLoS One 2015;10:e0137345.
27. Green MR, Kihira S, Liu CL, et al. Mutations in early follicular lymphoma progenitors are associated with suppressed antigen presentation. Proc Natl Acad Sci U S A 2015;112:E1116–25.
28. Bolden JE, Peart MJ, Johnstone RW. Anticancer activities of histone deacetylase inhibitors. Nat Rev Drug Discov 2006;5:769–84.
29. Bishton M, Kenealy M, Johnstone R, et al. Epigenetic targets in hematological malignancies: combination therapies with HDACis and demethylating agents. Expert Rev Anticancer Ther 2007;7:1439–49.
30. Devan J, Janikova A, Mraz M. New concepts in follicular lymphoma biology: from BCL2 to epigenetic regulators and non-coding RNAs. Semin Oncol 2018;45:291–302.
31. Piekarz RL, Robey RW, Zhan Z, et al. T-cell lymphoma as a model for the use of histone deacetylase inhibitors in cancer therapy: impact of depsipeptide on molecular markers, therapeutic targets, and mechanisms of resistance. Blood 2004;103:4636–43.
32. Kirschbaum M, Frankel P, Popplewell L, et al. Phase II study of vorinostat for treatment of relapsed or refractory indolent non-Hodgkin's lymphoma and mantle cell lymphoma. J Clin Oncol 2011;29:1198–203.
33. Ogura M, Ando K, Suzuki T, et al. A multicentre phase II study of vorinostat in patients with relapsed or refractory indolent B-cell non-Hodgkin lymphoma and mantle cell lymphoma. Br J Haematol 2014;165:768–76.

34. Chen R, Frankel P, Popplewell L, et al. A phase II study of vorinostat and rituximab for treatment of newly diagnosed and relapsed/refractory indolent non-Hodgkin lymphoma. Haematologica 2015;100:357–62.

35. Fouliard S, Robert R, Jacquet-Bescond A, et al. Pharmacokinetic/pharmacodynamic modelling-based optimisation of administration schedule for the histone deacetylase inhibitor abexinostat (S78454/PCI-24781) in phase I. Eur J Cancer 2013;49:2791–7.

36. Ribrag V, Kim WS, Bouabdallah R, et al. Safety and efficacy of abexinostat, a pan-histone deacetylase inhibitor, in non-Hodgkin lymphoma and chronic lymphocytic leukemia: results of a phase II study. Haematologica 2017;102:903–9.

37. Evens AM, Balasubramanian S, Vose JM, et al. A phase I/II multicenter, open-label study of the oral histone deacetylase inhibitor abexinostat in relapsed/refractory lymphoma. Clin Cancer Res 2016;22:1059–66.

38. Batlevi CL, Crump M, Andreadis C, et al. A phase 2 study of mocetinostat, a histone deacetylase inhibitor, in relapsed or refractory lymphoma. Br J Haematol 2017;178:434–41.

39. Bodor C, Grossmann V, Popov N, et al. EZH2 mutations are frequent and represent an early event in follicular lymphoma. Blood 2013;122:3165–8.

40. Knutson SK, Kawano S, Minoshima Y, et al. Selective inhibition of EZH2 by EPZ-6438 leads to potent antitumor activity in EZH2-mutant non-Hodgkin lymphoma. Mol Cancer Ther 2014;13:842–54.

41. Morschhauser F, Tilly H, Chaidos A, et al. Phase 2 Multicenter Study of Tazemetostat, an EZH2 Inhibitor, in Patients with Relapsed or Refractory Follicular Lymphoma. Blood 2019;134 (Supplement_1):123.

42. Danial NN, Korsmeyer SJ. Cell death: critical control points. Cell 2004;116:205–19.

43. Llambi F, Moldoveanu T, Tait SW, et al. A unified model of mammalian BCL-2 protein family interactions at the mitochondria. Mol Cell 2011;44:517–31.

44. Roberts AW, Seymour JF, Brown JR, et al. Substantial susceptibility of chronic lymphocytic leukemia to BCL2 inhibition: results of a phase I study of navitoclax in patients with relapsed or refractory disease. J Clin Oncol 2012;30:488–96.

45. Davids MS, Roberts AW, Seymour JF, et al. Phase I first-in-human study of venetoclax in patients with relapsed or refractory non-Hodgkin lymphoma. J Clin Oncol 2017;35:826–33.

46. McDonnell TJ, Korsmeyer SJ. Progression from lymphoid hyperplasia to high-grade malignant lymphoma in mice transgenic for the t(14; 18). Nature 1991;349:254–6.

47. Roulland S, Kelly RS, Morgado E, et al. t(14;18) Translocation: a predictive blood biomarker for follicular lymphoma. J Clin Oncol 2014;32:1347–55.

48. Gibbs D, Van Besien H, Regan S, et al. Combined EZH2 and BCL2 Inhibitors As Precision Therapy for Genetically Defined DLBCL Subtypes. Blood 2019;134 (Supplement_1):304

49. de Vos S, Swinnen LJ, Wang D, et al. Venetoclax, bendamustine, and rituximab in patients with relapsed or refractory NHL: a phase 1b dose-finding study. Ann Oncol 2018;29(9):1932–8.

50. Gobessi S, Laurenti L, Longo PG, et al. Inhibition of constitutive and BCR-induced Syk activation downregulates Mcl-1 and induces apoptosis in chronic lymphocytic leukemia B cells. Leukemia 2009;23:686–97.

51. Andorsky DJ, Kolibaba KS, Assouline S, et al. An open-label phase 2 trial of entospletinib in indolent non-Hodgkin lymphoma and mantle cell lymphoma. Br J Haematol 2019;184:215–22.

52. Yildiz M, Li H, Bernard D, et al. Activating STAT6 mutations in follicular lymphoma. Blood 2015;125:668–79.
53. Smith S, Munoz J, Stevens D, et al. Rapid and Durable Responses with the SYK/JAK Inhibitor Cerdulatinib in a Phase 2 Study in Relapsed/Refractory Follicular Lymphoma—Alone or in Combination with Rituximab. Blood 2019;134(Supplement_1):3981.
54. Advani A, Coiffier B, Czuczman MS, et al. Safety, pharmacokinetics, and preliminary clinical activity of inotuzumab ozogamicin, a novel immunoconjugate for the treatment of B-cell non-Hodgkin's lymphoma: results of a phase I study. J Clin Oncol 2010;28:2085–93.
55. Fayad L, Offner F, Smith MR, et al. Safety and clinical activity of a combination therapy comprising two antibody-based targeting agents for the treatment of non-Hodgkin lymphoma: results of a phase I/II study evaluating the immunoconjugate inotuzumab ozogamicin with rituximab. J Clin Oncol 2013;31:573–83.
56. Morschhauser F, Flinn IW, Advani R, et al. Polatuzumab vedotin or pinatuzumab vedotin plus rituximab in patients with relapsed or refractory non-Hodgkin lymphoma: final results from a phase 2 randomised study (ROMULUS). Lancet Haematol 2019;6:e254–65.
57. Advani RH, Flinn I, Sharman JP, et al. Two doses of polatuzumab vedotin (PoV, anti-CD79b antibody-drug conjugate) in patients (pts) with relapsed/refractory (RR) follicular lymphoma (FL): durable responses at lower dose level. J Clin Oncol 2015;33:8503.
58. Sehn LH, Kamdar M, Herrera AF, et al. Randomized phase 2 trial of polatuzumab vedotin (pola) with bendamustine and rituximab (BR) in relapsed/refractory (r/r) FL and DLBCL. J Clin Oncol 2018;36:7507.
59. Diefenbach C, Kahl B, Banerjee L, et al. Polatuzumab vedotin plus obinutuzumab and lenalidomide in patients with relapsed/refractory follicular lymphoma: primary analysis of the full efficacy population in a phase Ib/II trial. Blood 2019;134(Supplement_1):126.
60. Fowler N, Nastoupil L, Chin CK, et al. A Phase I/II Study of Lenalidomide Plus Obinutuzumab in Relapsed Indolent Lymphoma. Blood 2019;134(Supplement_1):348.
61. Witzig TE, Molina A, Gordon LI, et al. Long-term responses in patients with recurring or refractory B-cell non-Hodgkin lymphoma treated with yttrium 90 ibritumomab tiuxetan. Cancer 2007;109:1804–10.
62. Witzig TE, Flinn IW, Gordon LI, et al. Treatment with ibritumomab tiuxetan radioimmunotherapy in patients with rituximab-refractory follicular non-Hodgkin's lymphoma. J Clin Oncol 2002;20:3262–9.
63. Moustafa MA, Parrando R, Wiseman G, et al. Long-Term Outcome of Patients with Low-Grade Follicular Lymphoma Treated with Yttrium-90 Ibritumomab Tiuxetan: The Mayo Clinic Experience. Blood 2019;134(Supplement_1):2809.
64. Spiess C, Zhai Q, Carter PJ. Alternative molecular formats and therapeutic applications for bispecific antibodies. Mol Immunol 2015;67:95–106.
65. Bargou R, Leo E, Zugmaier G, et al. Tumor regression in cancer patients by very low doses of a T cell-engaging antibody. Science 2008;321:974–7.
66. Schuster SJ, Bartlett NL, Assouline S, et al. Mosunetuzumab Induces Complete Remissions in Poor Prognosis Non-Hodgkin Lymphoma Patients, Including Those Who Are Resistant to or Relapsing After Chimeric Antigen Receptor T-Cell (CAR-T) Therapies, and Is Active in Treatment through Multiple Lines. Blood 2019;134 (Supplement_1):6.
67. Morschhauser F, Carlo-Stella C, Offner F, et al. Dual CD20-Targeted Therapy With Concurrent CD20-TCB and Obinutuzumab Shows Highly Promising Clinical

Activity and Manageable Safety in Relapsed or Refractory B-Cell Non-Hodgkin Lymphoma: Preliminary Results From a Phase Ib Trial. Blood 2019;134(Supplement_1):1584.

68. Baliga R, Li J, Manlusoc M, et al. High Avidity IgM-Based CD20xCD3 Bispecific Antibody (IGM-2323) for Enhanced T-Cell Dependent Killing with Minimal Cytokine Release. Blood 2019;134 (Supplement_1):1574.

69. Morschhauser F, Ghosh N, Lossos I, et al. Efficacy and safety of obinutuzumab + lenalidomide + atezolizumab in patients with relapsed or refractory follicular lymphoma: primary analysis of a phase 1B/2 trial. Hematol Oncol 2019;37:113–4.

70. Zinzani PL, Topp MS, Yuen SL, et al. Phase 2 study of venetoclax plus rituximab or randomized ven plus bendamustine+rituximab (BR) versus BR in patients with relapsed/refractory follicular lymphoma: interim data. Blood 2016;128:617.

71. Bartlett NL, Sehn LH, Assouline SE, et al. Managing cytokine release syndrome (CRS) and neurotoxicity with step-fractionated dosing of mosunetuzumab in relapsed/refractory (R/R) B-cell non-Hodgkin lymphoma (NHL). J Clin Oncol 2019;37:7518.

72. Dickinson MJ, Morschhauser F, Iacoboni G, et al. CD20-TCB (RG6026), a novel "2:1" format T-cell-engaging bispecific antibody, induces complete remissions in relapsed/refractory B-cell non-Hodgkin's lymphoma. Hematol Oncol 2019; 37:92–3.

Early Progression of Follicular Lymphoma
Biology and Treatment

Jodi J. Lipof, MD*, Paul M. Barr, MD

KEYWORDS

- Follicular lymphoma • Early progression • POD24 • Early relapse

KEY POINTS

- A majority of patients with follicular lymphoma follow an indolent disease course, but a subset of patients experiences early progression and inferior survival.
- The biology of early progression involves the complex interaction between neoplastic cells and the tumor microenvironment.
- There are several clinicogenetic prognostic indices aimed at identifying high-risk patients at diagnosis, each with strengths and limitations.
- Optimal treatment at time of early progression remains to be determined and is the subject of ongoing clinical trials.
- This high-risk population should be a priority in clinical trial development for follicular lymphoma.

INTRODUCTION

Follicular lymphoma (FL) is the most common subtype of indolent non-Hodgkin lymphoma (iNHL), representing approximately 20% to 30% of cases and characterized by neoplastic germinal center B cells.[1] In approximately 90% of FL cases, neoplastic B cells harbor the t(14;18) (q32;q21) *IGH/BCL2* translocation, which develops as a result of errors during V(D)J recombination in the bone marrow and leads to overexpression of *BCL2*, an antiapoptotic protein.[2,3] This translocation also is detected in B cells of healthy individuals, highlighting that additional genetic and epigenetic alterations must occur for the development of FL.[4,5]

A majority of patients follow an indolent disease course with a relapsing and remitting pattern, leading to overall survival (OS) of upwards of 20 years.[6] Despite this favorable prognosis in a majority of patients, approximately 20% of patients experience early disease progression after initial treatment with chemoimmunotherapy and a

James P. Wilmot Cancer Institute, University of Rochester Medical Center, 601 Elmwood Avenue, Rochester, NY 14642, USA
* Corresponding author.
E-mail address: Jodi_Lipof@urmc.rochester.edu

Hematol Oncol Clin N Am 34 (2020) 757–769
https://doi.org/10.1016/j.hoc.2020.02.009
0889-8588/20/© 2020 Elsevier Inc. All rights reserved.

hemonc.theclinics.com

smaller subset of patients undergoes transformation to aggressive large cell lymphoma.[7–9]

EARLY PROGRESSING FOLLICULAR LYMPHOMA

The National LymphoCare Study (NLCS) is a prospective, observational study of approximately 2700 newly diagnosed FL patients. Casulo and colleagues[10] performed a large analysis of 588 of these patients treated with frontline rituximab, cyclophosphamide, doxorubicin, vincristine, and prednisone (R-CHOP). They found that approximately 20% of patients progress within 24 months of initial treatment and have inferior 5-year OS of 50% versus 90% in patients without early progression. This was validated in a pooled data set of 5453 patients from 13 large clinical trials by the Follicular Lymphoma Analysis of Surrogacy Hypothesis study, where early progression emerged as the most significant independent risk factor for inferior survival (5-y OS 87.5% in the 24 months of follow-up with no progression of disease or death due to progression of disease during that time [noPOD24] group vs 62% in the progression of disease within 24 months [POD24] group; *P<.0001*).[11] Inferior outcomes after bendamustine-based therapy have been demonstrated as well. A recent retrospective study by a British Columbia group showed 13% of patients treated with bendamustine and rituximab (BR) experienced POD24.[12] Although the rate of POD24 events appeared to be lower, they also found that a higher percentage of these patients had transformed disease at progression (76%). Event-free survival at 12 months was evaluated in 920 patients enrolled on the University of Iowa/Mayo Clinic Lymphoma SPORE Molecular Epidemiology Resource and again showed that early relapse after chemoimmunotherapy led to inferior outcomes.[13]

This high-risk, early progressing population has become a priority in FL research.[14] Several prognostic indices have been developed with the goal of identifying these patients prior to treatment, each with their own strengths and pitfalls. Several targeted, nonchemotherapeutic agents have shown promising activity and efficacy in this population, with tolerable side-effect profiles. Early identification of these patients and tailored treatment remain challenging, however, and have become priorities in clinical trial development for FL.

BIOLOGY OF EARLY PROGRESSING FOLLICULAR LYMPHOMA

FL B cells retain surface immunoglobulin despite the translocation of 1 allele leading to the pathognomonic t(14;18). They contain identical immunoglobulin heavy chain gene rearrangements, indicating that founder mutations that contribute to lymphomagenesis must take place after V(D)J recombination.[15] These t(14;18)+ cells are IgM+ and prone to reentering the germinal center repeatedly without undergoing class-switching like normal B cells, allowing them to accumulate secondary and tertiary genetic and epigenetic alterations that are necessary for the development of FL.[16]

Study of the mutational diversity between diagnostic and relapse specimens has aided in development of models for the genetic evolution of FL. One model describes early founder mutations that prolong the life of a premalignant clone, allowing for accumulation of additional driver mutations that lead to a malignant clone. Tertiary accelerator or passenger mutations may play an important role in relapse and progression by providing a selective advantage for malignant clones to proliferate and expand.[17] Whole-exome sequencing of serial tumor samples has revealed recurrently mutated genes, with a notable increase in chromatin-modification gene mutations, leading to epigenetic dysregulation.[18]

Sequencing efforts comparing diagnostic and relapsed lymphoma specimens have provided insights into the molecular differences in early progressing FL, demonstrating markedly different clonal dynamics compared with never progressing or later progressing patients and transformed FL.[19] Expectedly, there is a higher mutational burden that develops at progression and appears independent of the time interval between sampling. The expanded clones at transformation were rare or absent at diagnosis suggesting that predictors of transformation may be difficult to identify based on this work. The clonal architecture in cases of early progressing FL, however, was present at diagnosis and exhibited relative stability despite chemoimmunotherapy. Cases of early progression appear to harbor intrinsic chemoresistant properties at diagnosis whereas the transformation phenotype appears to be acquired over the course of the disease. This observation supports the development of a predictive model incorporating the molecular aberrations driving resistance and potentially guiding alternative therapy for such patients.

Microenvironment

Growing evidence has shown that the survival and proliferation of neoplastic FL cells depends heavily on interaction with surrounding non-neoplastic cells in the microenvironment. Dave and colleagues[20] created 2 distinct immunologic, gene expression signatures of non-neoplastic, tumor-infiltrating cells, which were associated with difference in progression-free survival (PFS) and OS. They showed that the gene expression profile of the microenvironment has an impact on disease course. Gene expression profile reflective of T-cell–restricted genes and macrophages was associated with more favorable outcomes, whereas a signature consistent with infiltration of macrophages, dendritic cells, or both was associated with less favorable outcomes.

The presence of regulatory T cells (Tregs) and the pattern in which they are distributed also have been shown of prognostic significance, enhancing tumor recognition and antitumoral immunoactivity.[21–23] In FL, the qualitative distribution of FOXP3$^+$ Tregs in a follicular versus perifollicular pattern has been associated with outcome. The presence of FOXP3$^+$ Tregs in a follicular pattern has been associated with inferior survival as well as increased risk of transformation.[24]

Programmed Cell Death Axis

Study of immune checkpoints has led to significant improvements in the understanding of intratumoral suppression of programmed cell death. Within the FL microenvironment, increased tumor-infiltrating lymphocytes with programmed cell death ligand 1 (PD-L1) expression is associated with favorable outcomes and decreased PD-L1$^+$ tumor-infiltrating lymphocytes associated with higher-grade disease and higher risk of transformation.[25] Tobin and colleagues[26] created tumor immune infiltration profiles to determine correlation with increased risk of POD24. Consistent with previous work, clinical outcomes within the patient cohorts correlated with intratumoral infiltration of immune cells. Low expression of PD-L2 (programmed cell death ligand 2), CD4, CD68, and tumor necrosis factor (TNF) α were associated with adverse outcomes. Of these markers, they found low PD-L2 expression to have the highest accuracy in predicting for POD24 and this was validated in 2 independent cohorts. Approximately 45% of patients with low PD-L2 expression experienced POD24 whereas only 16% to 25% ($P = .001$) of those with high PD-L2 experienced such events. They also performed sequencing and gene expression profiling on these specimens and found that the mutational profiles were similar regardless of immune infiltration level. This indicates that tumor biology and the tumor microenvironment are independent factors that influence disease course. Therefore, a model combining molecular features of the FL tumor cells as well as the microenvironment immune profile may further improve the ability to prospectively identify early progression of disease patients.

PROGNOSTIC INDICES

Several prognostic indices incorporating clinical and biologic factors have been developed to identify high-risk patients at diagnosis and predict survival. These include the Follicular Lymphoma International Prognostic Index (FLIPI), FLIPI2, m7-FLIPI, POD24-Prognostic Index (PI), and a 23-gene predictor (**Table 1**).

Follicular Lymphoma International Prognostic Index/Follicular Lymphoma International Prognostic Index 2

The most widely used prognostic model is the FLIPI, which includes 5 clinical factors: age (<60 or >60), Ann Arbor stages III–IV disease, hemoglobin (<12 g/dL or >12 g/dL), involved nodal areas (<4 or >4), and elevated lactate dehydrogenase (LDH).[27] Patients are divided into low risk, intermediate risk, and high risk, which were shown to be associated with differential 5-year OS rates of 91%, 78%, and 52%, respectively. This scoring system was developed in prerituximab era but remains relevant with modern chemoimmunotherapy.[28]

A second scoring system, the FLIPI2, was based on prospective analysis of patients treated with standard chemoimmunotherapy.[29] This prognostic index similarly combined laboratory and clinical factors: age, bone marrow involvement, hemoglobin, β_2-microglobulin, and longest diameter of the largest lymph node involved. The FLIPI2 divides patient into low-risk, intermediate-risk, and high-risk groups that result in 3-year PFS rates of 91%, 69%, and 51%, respectively. In comparison to the FLIPI, it seems to have more accuracy in prognostication but has limited ability to direct treatment decisions.[30]

m7-Follicular Lymphoma International Prognostic Index

The m7-FLIPI was developed with the goal of incorporating disease biology and clinical factors into a prognostic index that could predict survival with more accuracy. Pastore and colleagues[31] performed sequencing studies of 74 recurrently mutated genes in FL and found that the mutational status of 7 genes (EZH2, ARID1A, EP300, FOXO1, MEF2B, CREBBP, and CARD11) in combination with Eastern Cooperative Group Performance Status (ECOG PS) and FLIPI score were associated with outcome. This clinicopathologic model was predictive of failure-free survival (FFS). In the validation cohort, the high-risk m7-FLIPI group had a 5-year FFS of 25% versus 68% in the low-risk group (P<.0001). Approximately half of patients initially identified as high risk by FLIPI were recategorized as low risk by m7-FLIPI and seemed to have outcomes consistent with that reclassification.

In an investigation to prospectively determine the predictive utility for POD24, Vindi and colleagues[32] found that approximately half of the patients with POD24 were classified as low risk based on the m7-FLIPI, highlighting a major limitation of its predictive capacity for early progression. Jurinovic and colleagues[33] found that the m7-FLIPI was superior to the FLIPI at specifically predicting POD24 but that approximately 39% to 43% of patients initially classified as low risk had POD24 whereas 14% to 21% of those identified as high risk did not. Despite lack of early progression in approximately a fifth of the high-risk group, further analysis did confirm that they had inferior outcomes.

In the work by Kridel and colleagues,[19] discussed previously, 10 genes were more commonly mutated in patients with early progression than in patients with late

Table 1
Outcomes and progression of disease within 24 months prediction by prognostic index

Prognostic Index	Risk Factors	High Risk	Progression-Free Survival	Progression of Disease Within 24 Months Risk	Overall Survival
FLIPI[27]	Age>60 >4 nodal sites Elevated LDH Hemoglobin: <12 g/dL Stages III–IV	3–5	20% (5-y PFS) 39% (3-y PFS)[30]	OR 3.2 ($P = .035$) 33% (PPV)[33]	89% (3 y)[30] 35% (10 y)
FLIPI2[29]	Age>60 High β_2-microglobulin Bone marrow involvement Largest node >6 cm Hemoglobin <12 g/dL	3–5	39% (3-y PFS)[30]	N/A	89% (3 y)[30]
m7-FLIPI[31]	FLIPI ECOG PS Mutation status: EZH2, ARID1A, EP300, FOXO1, MEF2B, CREBBP, CARD11	>0.8	25% (5-y FFS)[31]	OR 4.8 ($P = .0052$) 48% (PPV)[33]	89% (5 y)
POD24-PI[33]	High-risk FLIPI ECOG PS Nonsilent mutations in EP300, FOXO1, and EZH2	>0.71	62% (2-y FFS) 36% (5-y FFS)	OR 4.3 ($P = .0051$) 40% (PPV)	48% (5 y)
23-gene predictor[34]	Gene expression profile signature	>1.075	26% (5-y PFS)[34]	38% (PPV)	N/A

Abbreviations: OR, odds ratio; PPV, positive predictive value.
   Data from Refs.[27,29–31,33,34]

progression or never progression, including *KMT2C*, *TP53*, *BTG1*, *MKI67*, *XBP1*, and *SOCS1*. Many of these are not included in the m7-FLIPI. Although this prognostic tool seems to have higher predictive value than the FLIPI alone, refinement is needed to accurately identify these patients who are at high risk of early progression.

Progression of Disease Within 24 Months–Prognostic Index

Using the same data sets as for the m7-FLIPI, Jurinovic and colleagues[33] developed an additional prognostic index called the POD24-PI, aimed at achieving a higher sensitivity for prediction of POD24. This index included several factors: ECOG PS, high-risk FLIPI, and nonsilent mutations in *EP300*, *FOXO1*, and *EZH2*. The POD24-PI was found more sensitive but less specific for predicting POD24 than the m7-FLIPI (sensitivity 78% vs 61%, respectively; specificity 67% vs 79%, respectively).

23-Gene Predictor

The Lymphoma Study Association group used gene expression profiling to create a 23-gene based model to predict PFS.[34] They examined 160 specimens from untreated patients with high–tumor burden FL enrolled in the phase III PRIMA trial and developed high-risk and low-risk gene profile groups. They found that 5-year PFS was 26% in the high-risk group and 73% in the low-risk group, and this was independent of FLIPI score. They also found that POD24 was 38% in the high-risk group and

19% in the low-risk group, indicating possible utility of the model in predicting early progression.

Together, the prognostic systems reliably stratify patient cohorts according to clinical outcomes. The genes identified as part of the clinicomolecular profiles, however, currently are not evaluated as part of standard practice, limiting use by treating physicians. Furthermore, prospective trials investigating a precision therapeutic approach are lacking. As such, further study is required to identify patients at risk for early progression and to direct therapy for this high-risk population.

MANAGEMENT OF EARLY RELAPSED FOLLICULAR LYMPHOMA
Chemoimmunotherapy

Because a majority of patients with high–tumor burden disease initially receive combination chemoimmunotherapy, early disease progression has been defined following induction strategies, such R-CHOP, R-CVP (Rituximab, cyclophosphamide, vincristine and prednisone), or BR.[9,35,36] No prospective data are available detailing outcomes using alternative chemoimmunotherapy regimens in patients experiencing POD24. In unselected relapsed refractory patients, R-CHOP resulted in an 85% response rate, including 30% complete responses and 3-year median PFS. As such, CHOP-like therapy is considered a valid treatment option for patients not previously treated with an anthracycline.

Anti-CD20 Monoclonal Antibodies in Early Progressors

Obinutuzumab is a glycoengineered type II anti-CD20 monoclonal antibody with enhanced antibody-dependent cellular toxicity and direct cytotoxicity.[37] The GADO-LIN study was a randomized phase III study that compared obinutuzumab and bendamustine to single-agent bendamustine in rituximab-refractory patients.[38] They found an improvement in median PFS of 29 months versus 14 months, respectively, which led to the Food and Drug Administration approval of obinutuzumab for the treatment of rituximab-refractory patients. The GALLIUM study was a randomized phase III trial that assigned patients to obinutuzumab-based or rituximab-based chemotherapy.[39] They found an improved PFS at 3 years with the obinutuzumab-based regimen compared with the rituximab-based regimen (80% vs 73%; $P = .0012$). A subset analysis of the GALLIUM study found that there were fewer POD24 events in patients in the obinutuzumab group compared with those in the rituximab group (incidence rate 10.1% vs 17.4%; $P = .0003$). Together, these data favor the use of obinutuzumab over rituximab in the high-risk POD24 group.

Immunomodulatory Agents

The combination of obinutuzumab and lenalidomide was studied in a single-arm phase II study (GALEN) of patients with relapsed and refractory FL.[40] Patients received the combination for six 28-day cycles followed by combination maintenance for 1 year and single-agent obinutuzumab maintenance for an additional year. The overall response rate (ORR) was 79% after induction with a complete response rate of 38% and 2-year PFS of 65%. In 24 patients who experienced POD24 after first-line chemoimmunotherapy, similar response rates (70%) and 2-year PFS of 62.5% were observed, suggesting similar efficacy in a chemoresistant group.

In the phase III AUGMENT study,[41] which investigated rituximab and lenalidomide (R^2) compared with rituximab and placebo in 358 relapsed iNHL patients, the POD24 FL subgroup had the same ORR of 80% with R^2 as the group without POD24 and a CR rate of 30% (vs 39%).[42] The median PFS in the POD24 group was

30.4 months, which surpasses the median PFS for this high-risk group after other regimens that have been studied in the early relapse setting. Importantly, they excluded rituximab-refractory patients and included patients only who would be appropriate for rituximab monotherapy at relapse, inherently selecting for a potentially lower-risk group.

The MAGNIFY trial is an ongoing phase IIIb study investigating maintenance with rituximab versus R^2 after 12-month induction with R^2 in relapsed/refractory FL. A post-induction analysis of patients with early relapse after initial treatment with R-chemotherapy showed an ORR of 48%, CR rate of 12%, and 1-year PFS of 45%, supporting the activity and tolerability in this high-risk, treatment-refractory group.[43]

Phosphatidylinositol 3-kinase Inhibitors

Phosphatidylinositol 3-kinase (PI3K) inhibition has been an attractive target for B-cell malignancies due to its critical role in signaling pathways that mediate cell proliferation, migration, and maturation. There are 4 isoforms (α, β, γ, and δ) that comprise the catalytic subunit of the enzyme. The γ and δ isoforms are preferentially expressed on hematopoietic cells whereas the α and β isoforms are present in many tissues. Inhibition of the δ isoform has been shown to mitigate malignant B-cell proliferation whereas inhibition of the γ isoform has been shown to play a role in blocking T-cell signaling within the tumor microenvironment.[44]

Idelalisib is a selective, reversible, and competitive oral PI3Kδ inhibitor that was approved for use in patients refractory to rituximab and an alkylating agent based on the results of a phase II trial.[45] In a retrospective post hoc analysis of this study, the POD24 FL group was found to have similar response rates and PFS to all FL patients on the study.[46] They had an ORR of 56.8% (vs 57% in all FL) with median duration of response (DOR) 11.8 (vs 12.5) months and median PFS of 11.1 (vs 11) months. Toxicities limiting its use and leading to early discontinuation include colitis, transaminitis, cutaneous toxicities, neutropenia, and opportunistic infections, including *Pneumocystis jirovecii.*

Duvelisib is another oral PI3K inhibitor, which targets both the δ and γ subunits.[47] In the phase II DYNAMO study, which investigated single-agent duvelisib in 129 heavily pretreated patients with iNHL, the FL group had an ORR of 42.2%, with median DOR 10 months and median PFS of 9.5 months.[48] In a subgroup analysis of the high-risk POD24 group, there was an ORR of 33% with median DOR 12.6 months and PFS of 8.2 months, again suggesting that it may have comparable efficacy and durability in the higher-risk group. Side-effect profile was similar to idelalisib but with lower rates of colitis and transaminitis.

The intravenous pan-class I *PI3K* inhibitor, copanlisib, was approved on the basis of a single-arm, phase II study that looked at 142 patients with relapsed and refractory iNHL.[49] Outcomes in the POD24 subgroup analysis were similar to all FL patients included on the trial.[50] ORR in this high-risk group was 60% (vs 59% in all FL), with median PFS of 11.3 (vs 11.2) months and median DOR of 14.9 (vs. 12.2) months. The side-effect profile of copanlisib was different from idelalisib and duvelisib, with higher rates of hypertension and hyperglycemia due to increased inhibition of the α isoform. Importantly, the POD24 group after initial treatment with R-CHOP had a complete response (CR) rate of 29%, suggesting that this might be a highly effective option in a chemoresistant group (**Table 2**).

Autologous Stem Cell Transplantation

For appropriate patients, salvage chemotherapy and high-dose chemotherapy with autologous stem cell transplantation (ASCT) remains an option associated with

Table 2
Response rates and efficacy of targeted agents in early progressing follicular lymphoma

Therapy	Overall Response Rate (%)	Progression-Free Survival	Duration of Response (mo)	Overall Survival
(R²)[42,43]	80,48	30.4 mo (median) 50% (1 y)	NA	NA
Lenalidomide and obinutuzumab[40]	70	62.5% (2 y)	NA	82.8% (2 y)
Idelalisib[46]	57	11 mo (median)	11.8	NA
Duvelisib[48]	33	8.2 mo (median)	12.6	NA
Copanlisib[50]	60	11.3 mo (median)	14.9	42.6 mo (median)

Abbreviation: NA, not available.
Data from Refs.[40,42,43,46,48,50]

prolonged remissions in FL. In a retrospective study by the Grupo Español de Linfomas y Trasplantes de Médula Ósea (GELTAMO), patients who underwent ASCT had a medians PFS and OS of 9.7 years and 21.3 years, respectively.[51] They also found that the PFS curves plateau after 16 years for patients who underwent ASCT in CR, suggesting that a subset of these patients might be cured. Like others before, they found that those who were treated in CR1 or CR2 had excellent outcomes, confirming that ASCT provides most benefit earlier in the disease course.[52]

Casulo and colleagues[53] specifically identified high-risk patients with early treatment failure within 2 years of initial treatment with chemoimmunotherapy and analyzed data from the NLCS and Center for International Blood and Marrow Transplant Research (CIBMTR). They found improved 5-year OS in patients who underwent ASCT within 1 year of treatment failure compared with patients who did not undergo ASCT (73% vs 60%; $P = .05$), supporting use of ASCT for eligible patients experiencing early FL progression.

Taken together, the available data suggest that alternative strategies may partially overcome the chemoresistant phenotype of early FL progression. This supports the use of high-dose chemotherapy and autologous stem cell rescue in young fitter patients while focusing on targeted agents and second-generation anti-CD20 antibodies in older patients. Ongoing clinical trials are attempting to investigate this further. Conducted through the National Clinical Trials Network, S1608 is a randomized phase II trial enrolling POD24 patients (NCT03269669). Participants receive lenalidomide, the PI3K inhibitor umbralisib, or additional chemotherapy, in conjunction with obinutuzumab (**Fig. 1**). Aimed at defining the optimal induction regimen, patients subsequently can pursue high-dose chemotherapy consolidation if needed. Additional broader clinical trials continue to investigate novel therapeutics, including cellular therapy and molecularly targeted agents.

Allogeneic Stem Cell Transplantation

Smith and colleagues[54] performed a retrospective analysis of the CIBMTR data comparing outcomes in patients with early treatment failure within 2 years of initial chemoimmunotherapy undergoing either ASCT or allogeneic stem cell transplantation (alloSCT) with an HLA matched sibling donor (MSD) or matched unrelated donor (MUD). Although relapse rates were lower with alloSCT (MSD 31% and MUD 23%)

S1608: Randomized Phase II Trial in Early Progressing or Refractory Follicular Lymphoma

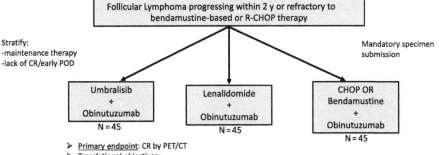

Fig. 1. Design of the SWOG 1608 (S1608) trial in early progressing or refractory FL.

than with ASCT (58%; $P<.0001$), 5-year OS rates were comparable between ASCT and MSD alloSCT (70% vs 73%, respectively) but lower in patients undergoing MUD alloSCT (49%; $P = .008$). Nonrelapse mortality was lowest in the ASCT group (5%) and higher in patients undergoing MSD alloSCT or MUD alloSCT (17% and 33%, respectively; $P<.001$). These data suggest that ASCT and MSD alloSCT are reasonable options for patients experiencing early progression.

SUMMARY

Although a vast majority of FL patients follow an indolent disease course, there is a subset of patients who experience early progression or transformation resulting in inferior survival. Although the molecular drivers of early progression have yet to be dissected, early studies support ongoing investigations aimed at identifying these patients at diagnosis. Several prognostic models have been evaluated in this regard. Thus far, the m7-FLIPI appears to exhibit the highest accuracy for prediction of early progression but remains limited in its sensitivity. These clinicogenetic models still require prospective investigation on a large scale to determine their utility in predicting early progressors and other patients at risk of inferior survival. Given the variety of treatment options available in the frontline and relapse settings, predictor biomarkers will require validation in patients treated with different induction strategies going forward. Clinical trials investigating the optimal approach in these patients in the era of novel therapeutics are absolutely essential. Whenever possible, these high-risk patients should be treated in the context of a clinical trial given their historically poor outcomes.

DISCLOSURE

P.M. Barr—advisory or consulting role: Pharmacyclics, AbbVie, Gilead, Seattle Genetics, Celgene, Genentech, Verastem, MorphoSys, and AstraZeneca. J.J. Lipof—nothing to disclose.

REFERENCES

1. Swerdlow SH, Campo E, Pileri SA, et al. The 2016 revision of the World Health Organization classification of lymphoid neoplasms. Blood 2016;127(20):2375–90.
2. Rowley JD. Chromosome studies in the non-Hodgkin's lymphomas: the role of the 14;18 translocation. J Clin Oncol 1988;6(5):919–25.
3. Tsujimoto Y, Cossman J, Jaffe E, et al. Involvement of the bcl-2 gene in human follicular lymphoma. Science 1985;228(4706):1440–3.
4. Summers KE, Goff LK, Wilson AG, et al. Frequency of the Bcl-2/IgH rearrangement in normal individuals: implications for the monitoring of disease in patients with follicular lymphoma. J Clin Oncol 2001;19(2):420–4.
5. Schmitt C, Balogh B, Grundt A, et al. The bcl-2/IgH rearrangement in a population of 204 healthy individuals: occurrence, age and gender distribution, breakpoints, and detection method validity. Leuk Res 2006;30(6):745–50.
6. Tan D, Horning SJ, Hoppe RT, et al. Improvements in observed and relative survival in follicular grade 1-2 lymphoma during 4 decades: the Stanford University experience. Blood 2013;122(6):981–7.
7. Mozessohn L, Cheung MC, Crump M, et al. Chemoimmunotherapy resistant follicular lymphoma: predictors of resistance, association with transformation and prognosis. Leuk Lymphoma 2014;55(11):2502–7.
8. Bachy E, Seymour JF, Feugier P, et al. Sustained progression-free survival benefit of rituximab maintenance in patients with follicular lymphoma: long-term results of the PRIMA study. J Clin Oncol 2019;37(31):2815–24.
9. Press OW, Unger JM, Rimsza LM, et al. Phase III randomized intergroup trial of CHOP plus rituximab compared with CHOP chemotherapy plus (131)iodine-tositumomab for previously untreated follicular non-Hodgkin lymphoma: SWOG S0016. J Clin Oncol 2013;31(3):314–20.
10. Casulo C, Byrtek M, Dawson KL, et al. Early relapse of follicular lymphoma after rituximab plus cyclophosphamide, doxorubicin, vincristine, and prednisone defines patients at high risk for death: an analysis from the National LymphoCare Study. J Clin Oncol 2015;33(23):2516–22.
11. Casulo C, Le-Rademacher J, Dixon J, et al. Validation of POD24 as a robust early clinical endpoint of poor survival in follicular lymphoma: results from the Follicular Lymphoma Analysis of Surrogacy Hypothesis (FLASH) investigation using individual data from 5,453 patients on 13 clinical trials. Blood 2017; 130(Supplement 1):412.
12. Freeman CL, Kridel R, Moccia AA, et al. Early progression after bendamustine-rituximab is associated with high risk of transformation in advanced stage follicular lymphoma. Blood 2019;134(9):761–4.
13. Maurer MJ, Bachy E, Ghesquieres H, et al. Early event status informs subsequent outcome in newly diagnosed follicular lymphoma. Am J Hematol 2016;91(11): 1096–101.
14. Maddocks K, Barr PM, Cheson BD, et al. Recommendations for Clinical Trial Development in Follicular Lymphoma. J Natl Cancer Inst 2017;109(3):255.
15. Irish JM, Czerwinski DK, Nolan GP, et al. Altered B-cell receptor signaling kinetics distinguish human follicular lymphoma B cells from tumor-infiltrating nonmalignant B cells. Blood 2006;108(9):3135–42.
16. Sungalee S, Mamessier E, Morgado E, et al. Germinal center reentries of BCL2-overexpressing B cells drive follicular lymphoma progression. J Clin Invest 2014; 124(12):5337–51.

17. Green MR, Gentles AJ, Nair RV, et al. Hierarchy in somatic mutations arising during genomic evolution and progression of follicular lymphoma. Blood 2013; 121(9):1604–11.

18. Green MR, Kihira S, Liu CL, et al. Mutations in early follicular lymphoma progenitors are associated with suppressed antigen presentation. Proc Natl Acad Sci U S A 2015;112(10):E1116–25.

19. Kridel R, Chan FC, Mottok A, et al. Histological transformation and progression in follicular lymphoma: a clonal evolution study. PLoS Med 2016;13(12):e1002197.

20. Dave SS, Wright G, Tan B, et al. Prediction of survival in follicular lymphoma based on molecular features of tumor-infiltrating immune cells. N Engl J Med 2004;351(21):2159–69.

21. Sakaguchi S, Setoguchi R, Yagi H, et al. Naturally arising Foxp3-expressing CD25+CD4+ regulatory T cells in self-tolerance and autoimmune disease. Curr Top Microbiol Immunol 2006;305:51–66.

22. Nishikawa H, Jager E, Ritter G, et al. CD4+ CD25+ regulatory T cells control the induction of antigen-specific CD4+ helper T cell responses in cancer patients. Blood 2005;106(3):1008–11.

23. Heier I, Hofgaard PO, Brandtzaeg P, et al. Depletion of CD4+ CD25+ regulatory T cells inhibits local tumour growth in a mouse model of B cell lymphoma. Clin Exp Immunol 2008;152(2):381–7.

24. Farinha P, Al-Tourah A, Gill K, et al. The architectural pattern of FOXP3-positive T cells in follicular lymphoma is an independent predictor of survival and histologic transformation. Blood 2010;115(2):289–95.

25. Carreras J, Lopez-Guillermo A, Roncador G, et al. High numbers of tumor-infiltrating programmed cell death 1-positive regulatory lymphocytes are associated with improved overall survival in follicular lymphoma. J Clin Oncol 2009; 27(9):1470–6.

26. Tobin JWD, Keane C, Gunawardana J, et al. Progression of Disease Within 24 Months in Follicular Lymphoma Is Associated With Reduced Intratumoral Immune Infiltration. J Clin Oncol 2019;37(34):3300–9.

27. Solal-Celigny P, Roy P, Colombat P, et al. Follicular lymphoma international prognostic index. Blood 2004;104(5):1258–65.

28. Buske C, Hoster E, Dreyling M, et al. The Follicular Lymphoma International Prognostic Index (FLIPI) separates high-risk from intermediate- or low-risk patients with advanced-stage follicular lymphoma treated front-line with rituximab and the combination of cyclophosphamide, doxorubicin, vincristine, and prednisone (R-CHOP) with respect to treatment outcome. Blood 2006;108(5):1504–8.

29. Federico M, Bellei M, Marcheselli L, et al. Follicular lymphoma international prognostic index 2: a new prognostic index for follicular lymphoma developed by the international follicular lymphoma prognostic factor project. J Clin Oncol 2009; 27(27):4555–62.

30. Arcaini L, Merli M, Passamonti F, et al. Validation of follicular lymphoma international prognostic index 2 (FLIPI2) score in an independent series of follicular lymphoma patients. Br J Haematol 2010;149(3):455–7.

31. Pastore A, Jurinovic V, Kridel R, et al. Integration of gene mutations in risk prognostication for patients receiving first-line immunochemotherapy for follicular lymphoma: a retrospective analysis of a prospective clinical trial and validation in a population-based registry. Lancet Oncol 2015;16(9):1111–22.

32. Vindi J, Kridel R, Staiger AM, et al. A clinicogenetic risk model (m7-FLIPI) prospectively identifies one-half of patients with early disease progression of follicular lymphoma after first-line immunochemotherapy. Blood 2015;126(23):333.

33. Jurinovic V, Kridel R, Staiger AM, et al. Clinicogenetic risk models predict early progression of follicular lymphoma after first-line immunochemotherapy. Blood 2016;128(8):1112–20.

34. Huet S, Tesson B, Jais JP, et al. A gene-expression profiling score for prediction of outcome in patients with follicular lymphoma: a retrospective training and validation analysis in three international cohorts. Lancet Oncol 2018;19(4):549–61.

35. Rummel MJ, Niederle N, Maschmeyer G, et al. Bendamustine plus rituximab versus CHOP plus rituximab as first-line treatment for patients with indolent and mantle-cell lymphomas: an open-label, multicentre, randomised, phase 3 non-inferiority trial. Lancet 2013;381(9873):1203–10.

36. Lansigan F, Barak I, Pitcher B, et al. The prognostic significance of PFS24 in follicular lymphoma following firstline immunotherapy: A combined analysis of 3 CALGB trials. Cancer Med 2019;8(1):165–73.

37. Mossner E, Brunker P, Moser S, et al. Increasing the efficacy of CD20 antibody therapy through the engineering of a new type II anti-CD20 antibody with enhanced direct and immune effector cell-mediated B-cell cytotoxicity. Blood 2010;115(22):4393–402.

38. Sehn LH, Chua N, Mayer J, et al. Obinutuzumab plus bendamustine versus bendamustine monotherapy in patients with rituximab-refractory indolent non-Hodgkin lymphoma (GADOLIN): a randomised, controlled, open-label, multicentre, phase 3 trial. Lancet Oncol 2016;17(8):1081–93.

39. Marcus R, Seymour JF, Hiddemann W. Obinutuzumab treatment of follicular lymphoma. N Engl J Med 2017;377(26):2605–6.

40. Morschhauser F, Le Gouill S, Feugier P, et al. Obinutuzumab combined with lenalidomide for relapsed or refractory follicular B-cell lymphoma (GALEN): a multicentre, single-arm, phase 2 study. Lancet Haematol 2019;6(8):e429–37.

41. Leonard JP, Trneny M, Izutsu K, et al. AUGMENT: a phase III study of lenalidomide plus rituximab versus placebo plus rituximab in relapsed or refractory indolent lymphoma. J Clin Oncol 2019;37(14):1188–99.

42. Leonard J, Trneny M, Izutsu K, et al. Augment phase III study: lenalidomide/rituximab (R2) improved efficacy over rituximab/placebo in relapsed/refractory follicular patients irrespective of POD24 status. Hematol Oncol 2019;37(S2):114–5.

43. Andorsky DJ, Yacoub A, Melear JM, et al. Phase IIIb randomized study of lenalidomide plus rituximab (R2) followed by maintenance in relapsed/refractory NHL: Analysis of patients with double-refractory or early relapsed follicular lymphoma (FL). J Clin Oncol 2017;35(15_suppl):7502.

44. Courtney KD, Corcoran RB, Engelman JA. The PI3K pathway as drug target in human cancer. J Clin Oncol 2010;28(6):1075–83.

45. Gopal AK, Kahl BS, de Vos S, et al. PI3Kdelta inhibition by idelalisib in patients with relapsed indolent lymphoma. N Engl J Med 2014;370(11):1008–18.

46. Gopal AK, Kahl BS, Flowers CR, et al. Idelalisib is effective in patients with high-risk follicular lymphoma and early relapse after initial chemoimmunotherapy. Blood 2017;129(22):3037–9.

47. Gyori D, Chessa T, Hawkins PT, et al. Class (I) phosphoinositide 3-kinases in the tumor microenvironment. Cancers (Basel) 2017;9(3) [pii:E24].

48. Flinn IW, Miller CB, Ardeshna KM, et al. DYNAMO: a phase II study of duvelisib (IPI-145) in patients with refractory indolent non-hodgkin lymphoma. J Clin Oncol 2019;37(11):912–22.

49. Dreyling M, Morschhauser F, Bouabdallah K, et al. Phase II study of copanlisib, a PI3K inhibitor, in relapsed or refractory, indolent or aggressive lymphoma. Ann Oncol 2017;28(9):2169–78.

50. Dreyling M, Santoro A, Leppä S, et al. Efficacy and safety in high-risk relapsed or refractory indolent follicular lymphoma patients treated with copanlisib. Hematol Oncol 2019;37(S2):387–9.
51. Jimenez-Ubieto A, Grande C, Caballero D, et al. Autologous stem cell transplantation for follicular lymphoma: favorable long-term survival irrespective of pre-transplantation rituximab exposure. Biol Blood Marrow Transplant 2017;23(10): 1631–40.
52. Kothari J, Peggs KS, Bird A, et al. Autologous stem cell transplantation for follicular lymphoma is of most benefit early in the disease course and can result in durable remissions, irrespective of prior rituximab exposure. Br J Haematol 2014; 165(3):334–40.
53. Casulo C, Friedberg JW, Ahn KW, et al. Autologous transplantation in follicular lymphoma with early therapy failure: a National LymphoCare Study and Center for International Blood and Marrow Transplant Research Analysis. Biol Blood Marrow Transplant 2018;24(6):1163–71.
54. Smith SM, Godfrey J, Ahn KW, et al. Autologous transplantation versus allogeneic transplantation in patients with follicular lymphoma experiencing early treatment failure. Cancer 2018;124(12):2541–51.

The Biological Basis of Histologic Transformation

Emil A. Kumar, BA, BM, BCh[a],*, Jessica Okosun, MB, BChir, PhD[b],
Jude Fitzgibbon, BA, PhD[a]

KEYWORDS

- Follicular • Lymphoma • Transformation • Genomics

KEY POINTS

- Histologic transformation of follicular lymphoma represents the leading cause of follicular lymphoma-related mortality, although cumulative incidence has decreased to less than 10% with anti-CD20 therapy.
- No single biological event is specific for histologic transformation, but recurrent genomic aberrations include dysregulation of cell cycle control and DNA damage response through *CDKN2A/B* and *TP53* loss, *MYC* activation, and nuclear factor-κB–associated mutations.
- Molecular heterogeneity may partly reflect the underlying clinical heterogeneity, with outcomes worse for histologic transformation after multiple lines of therapy versus treatment-naïve cases.
- Histologic transformation occurs predominantly by divergent, nonlinear clonal evolution from a putative common progenitor cell.
- An improved understanding of the interplay between genetic, epigenetic, and immune microenvironmental factors may enable discovery of novel diagnostic and therapeutic biomarkers.

INTRODUCTION

Histologic transformation (HT) of follicular lymphoma (FL) to a clonally related aggressive B-cell lymphoma represents a significant step-change in the clinical disease trajectory of a patient with FL. Although the addition of anti-CD20 therapy with rituximab has seen both the reduced cumulative incidence of transformation (from approximately 30% to approximately 8%–15%),[1–6] and improved outcomes for those who do transform,[2–4,7] transformation still represents the leading cause of FL-related

a Centre for Cancer Genomics and Computational Biology, Barts Cancer Institute, Queen Mary University of London, Charterhouse Square, London EC1M 6BQ, UK; b Centre for Haemato-Oncology, Barts Cancer Institute, Queen Mary University of London, Charterhouse Square, London EC1M 6BQ, UK
* Corresponding author.
E-mail address: e.a.kumar@qmul.ac.uk
Twitter: @fitzgi02 (J.F.)

mortality.[8] Hence, considerable interest remains in understanding the biological correlates of this critical disease event, which may translate into tools to improve prediction, detection and treatment.

DEFINITION

The gold standard for the identification of HT remains an adequate tissue biopsy, although cases diagnosed by consensus clinical criteria seemed to have equivalent outcomes to their histologically confirmed counterparts, at least in the prerituximab era.[3] HT is characterized morphologically by large cell effacement of the lymph node follicular architecture. The increased proportion of large B cells is key to the diagnosis of HT, with variable levels of diffuse involvement without large cell transformation also possible in indolent FL.[9] Although the immunophenotype of the mature germinal center (GC) B cell with aberrant BCL2 expression is typically preserved, there may be antigenic drift, including CD10 loss or new MUM1 positivity.[10] HT may be present at diagnosis itself, with a composite diagnosis referring to low-grade and high-grade disease occurring within the same biopsy, and discordant diagnosis to low-grade and high-grade disease at different sites. Outcomes for these entities are typically comparable with de novo diffuse large B-cell lymphoma (DLBCL),[6,11] albeit with an additional ongoing risk of indolent relapse.[12]

Using the World Health Organization classification criteria,[9,13] most HT cases constitute a diagnosis of DLBCL, although cases of high-grade B-cell lymphoma (with MYC and BCL2 and/or BCL6 translocations; or not otherwise specified with Burkitt-like features), and even B-lymphoblastic leukemia/lymphoma are also seen.[14–17]

Histologic grading in FL is defined by the proportion of small centrocytic and larger centroblastic B cells, with grade 3 disease consisting of more than 15 centroblasts per high power field, and grade 3B distinguished from grade 3A by its complete lack of centrocytes.[9,13] It is debated whether grade 3 disease predicts transformation,[16,18,19] with interobserver variability[20] and relatively small numbers of grade 3 cases potentially confounding factors. A grade 1 to 3A versus 3B dichotomy has been proposed, with grade 3A disease often co-occurring with and sharing immunohistochemical features with grade 1 to 2 disease,[21–24] whereas by contrast the rarer grade 3B entity, which frequently co-occurs with DLBCL[21,23,24] and is treated as such, is typically enriched for features including t(14;18)/CD10 negativity, and MUM1/IRF positivity,[21,23–25] suggesting a genuine biological distinction. Intriguingly in this regard, however, Horn and colleagues[24] recently reaffirmed the distinction between FL grades 1 to 3A and 3B in their immunohistochemical/translocation profiles, but unexpectedly discovered that 3A and 3B disease shared a closely related gene expression profile, intermediate to that of grades 1 and 2 FL and DLBCL.

CHALLENGES IN STUDYING HISTOLOGIC TRANSFORMATION BIOLOGY

Several challenges have faced researchers of HT biology. The available pool of archival tissue is limited, particularly when seeking paired low-grade and transformed biopsies, and this lack is further compounded by frequent exclusion of HT cases from both FL and DLBCL clinical trials. There is considerable heterogeneity with respect to the range of prior therapies received before HT. Although Rusconi and colleagues[11] recently described an inverse relationship between number of therapy lines before transformation, and subsequent overall survival (**Fig. 1**), transformation is typically—and perhaps erroneously—considered as a single entity in biological studies to create adequately sized patient cohorts. It seems plausible that the poor outcomes for

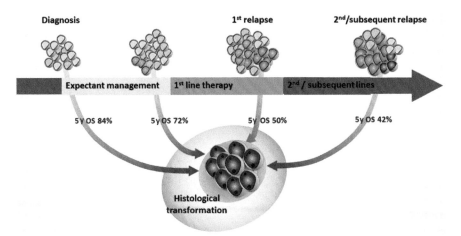

Fig. 1. The heterogeneity in clinical routes to HT. Although the various clinical routes to transformation are histologically indistinguishable, differences in outcomes likely reflect important heterogeneity in underlying biology. Five-year overall survival (OS) rates are presented. (*Data from* Rusconi C., Anastasia A., Chiarenza A., et al. Outcome of transformed follicular lymphoma worsens according to the timing of transformation and to the number of previous therapies. A retrospective multicenter study on behalf of Fondazione Italiana Linfomi (FIL). Br J Haematol 2019;185(4):713–7. Doi: 10.1111/bjh.15816.)

transformation after chemotherapy relative to treatment-naïve HT[5,11] reflect important biological features in the former group that may be more akin to relapsed/refractory DLBCL. Finally, the propensity for prospective clinical trials to report progression-free survival rather than documenting rates of transformation and low-grade progression separately, limits our ability to understand the impact of different treatment modalities on transformation risk; indeed, recent retrospective analyses indicate that rituximab decreases HT incidence[7] and that bendamustine may decrease early low-grade progression without impacting on transformation rate.[26] The consideration of such treatment-specific effects on HT evolution may in turn shape the direction of future biological study.

RECURRENT GENETIC LESIONS ASSOCIATED WITH HISTOLOGIC TRANSFORMATION

The greatest strides in the description of the biology of FL transformation have occurred at the level of genomic aberrations and evolution, particularly since the advent of next-generation sequencing (NGS) technologies. The examined cohorts of sequential FL-HT biopsies have, however, typically preceded or bridged the rituximab era. The crucial insights gained, although furthering our understanding of HT, may need to be revisited in the context of modern therapy algorithms, albeit with the obvious limitations of a narrowed pool of cases and an evolving treatment landscape.

Studies have pointed to an increased genomic complexity and mutational burden at transformation,[27,28] as might be expected from the transformation-associated derailing of DNA repair and cell cycle control mechanisms, within the permissive genomic instability of the GC environment. Activation-induced cytidine deaminase–driven aberrant somatic hypermutation (aSHM) is considered increased at transformation within targets including *MYC*, *PAX5*, *RhoH/TTF*, and *PIM1*.[27,29] It is unclear to what extent there is an acceleration of the aSHM process as opposed to a continuing exposure to the GC reaction,[29] and indeed the specific nature and extent of the role of the aSHM in transformation remains untested functionally. It is notable, however, in this regard that targets of aSHM include several transformation-associated candidates, and that a higher baseline activation-induced cytidine deaminase expression has been linked to an increased transformation risk.[30]

Specific structural chromosomal abnormalities need recognition, and associate with increased transformation risk at diagnosis, including loss affecting 1p, 6q, and 17p,[31,32] genomic regions that notably contain tumor suppressors *TNFRSF14*, *TNFAIP3* and, *TP53* respectively, whereas gains of chromosome 2, 3q, and 5 also predict for HT.[33] Lesions enriched at transformation itself include chromosomal gains of 7, 8, and 21, as well as gains of 1q, 6p, 9q, and 17q, and losses of 6q and 17p,[34] although these events are not uniquely specific to the transformation phase alone, also occurring in pretransformation samples at lower incidence. We have to be mindful, also, that these studies predate the use of rituximab and the significant reduction in HT rate, and need up-to-date validation.

Cell Cycle and DNA Damage Response Dysregulation

Among the commonest genetic lesions linked to transformation are those associated with proteins involved in DNA damage response and cell cycle regulation, echoing abnormalities associated with disease aggressiveness in DLBCL and other tumor types. RB and p53 pathway dysregulation through *CDKN2A/B* loss is frequent, with a particular prominence of biallelic loss at transformation.[27,34,35] *TP53* is also recurrently disrupted in HT by mutation and/or deletion, occurring in approximately 20% to 30% cases.[27,28,36] Indeed, the apparent convergence on the DNA damage response is underlined by the approximately two-thirds of transformed cases with biallelic loss of *CDKN2A/B* and/or *TP53*.[27] However, *TP53* loss also seems to represent a nonspecific indicator of poor risk disease, also occurring in nontransformed FL—particularly in cases who experience early progression.[28] Expression of negative p53 regulator, MDM2, is frequently increased at transformation, and may be more specific.[34,37] The master GC cell cycle regulator and proto-onocogene *MYC* is dysregulated by translocation, amplification, and/or aSHM in approximately 40% of HT,[27] with enrichment of MYC-regulated gene expression seen at transformation in at least a proportion of cases.[38,39] Musilova and colleagues[40] performed microRNA (miR) profiling of serial FL-HT biopsies, and found 5 miRs enriched at transformation, including miR-150. They propose an MYC/miR-150/FOXP1 axis whereby MYC overexpression induces higher miR-150 levels, in turn leading to greater expression of FOXP1: a transcription factor itself involved in B-cell development and associated with the ABC subtype of DLBCL and poor outcomes in both DLBCL and FL.[40,41]

Other Genomic Events

Other important processes recurrently implicated in transformation include nuclear factor (NF)-κB activation with *REL* amplification, mutation/loss of *TNFAIP3* and *MYD88* mutation,[34,37] and immune evasion through mutation/deletion of HLA class I components (most notably *B2M*) and *CD58*.[27,34] The block on terminal differentiation appears to be reinforced with increased *BCL6* translocation rate/copy number,[34,42] whereas enrichment of the *EBF1* mutation at transformation also seems to further dysregulate B-cell differentiation.[28,37]

Overall, despite the recurring trends observed, the molecular heterogeneity of HT is considerable, which may partly reflect the clinical heterogeneity in the sampled cases as discussed elsewhere in this article. This factor, and the variable presence of HT-associated aberrations in low-grade tumors (albeit at lower frequency), have hampered the definition of a transformation-specific genomic signature. Indeed the limitations in the sensitivity and specificity of these genomic events for HT highlight the importance of parallel investigative approaches, including gene expression profiling and immune microenvironment characterization, to paint a complete picture of transformation biology. Ultimately, HT may be best characterized as several discrete disease entities rather than one, echoing the current efforts to molecularly reclassify de novo DLBCL.[43–45]

CLONAL EVOLUTION

Studies examining sequential FL-HT biopsies have been pivotal in unraveling the clonal dynamics of FL transformation, with our increasing depth of understanding mirroring the advances in genomic technologies. Early studies confirmed that FL tumors and subsequent HT episodes are clonally related, with conservation of t(14;18) major breakpoint region and SHM patterns.[33,46,47] However, studies examining SHM patterns, copy neutral loss of heterozygosity, and copy number alterations consistently showed that most sequential cases harbor abnormalities unique to the initial FL episode, as well as new HT-unique and FL/HT-shared aberrations.[33,34,47,48] This finding points to disease episodes resulting from divergent evolution from a putative common progenitor cell (CPC), which evades eradication by treatment, and separately acquires secondary hits. Wang and colleagues[12] recently reported that of DLBCL patients experiencing late relapse (>2 years), around one-quarter of these recurrences consisted of indolent disease (>90% with FL). This suggests that CPC-seeded events may occur in the reverse order, that is, DBLCL followed by FL, although of course an unknown proportion of these cases may reflect a failure to detect discordant disease present at diagnosis. Meanwhile, case reports of donor-derived FL, whereby stem cell donors and recipients developed clonally related FL or HT several years after transplantation, confirms the ability of a CPC reservoir able to separately seed both FL and HT events at long latency.[47,49] Efforts to isolate and characterize this CPC population may thus ultimately unlock therapeutic opportunities for disease cure.

Crucially, NGS technologies have allowed genome-wide study of sequential FL-HT biopsies, and have confirmed the predominance of divergent clonal evolution (**Fig. 2**), with only a minority of cases showing a linear evolution consisting of direct acquisition of additional genetic hits by the dominant FL clone.[27,28,37] Examination of the shared mutations between FL and HT episodes allows a description of the inferred CPC, with a particular predominance of epigenetic mutations (*CREBBP*, *KMT2D*, and *EZH2*) within the ancestral clone.[27,37] Kridel and colleagues[28] used ultrasensitive mutation detection to construct high-resolution phylogenetic trees, and described contrasting clonal dynamics between HT and low-grade progression. Transformation typically displayed positive selection and dramatic expansion of subclones either undetectable or present at low levels (as low as 0.02%) in the initial FL biopsy, whereas low-grade progression was characterized by expansion of preexisting subclones. Somewhat surprisingly, the dramatic clonal dynamics seen with HT occurred largely independently of prior immunochemotherapy or time to transformation.

One area of incomplete understanding but considerable interest is the role of epigenetic mutations, including *KMT2D, CREBBP, EZH2*, and *EP300*, in HT. These lesions are well-established as early, disease-initiating events in low-grade FL,[27,28,37,50,51] and the lymphoma-promoting functional consequences of individual epimutations have emerged, such as the GC expansion and terminal differentiation block induced by KMT2D loss,[52,53] and downregulation of MHC class I/II seen with *CREBBP*[51] and *EZH2*[54] mutations. However, the degree to which the transcriptional reprogramming

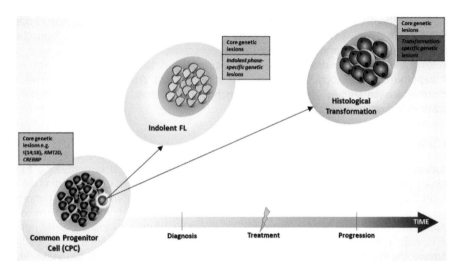

Fig. 2. Divergent clonal evolution underpins HT. An illustrative case of successive indolent FL and HT episodes. The majority of cases progress by sequential divergent clonal evolution from an inferred CPC, as evidenced by the presence of indolent phase-specific, as well as shared and transformation-specific genetic aberrations.

they induce is required for the evolution and maintenance of the aggressive HT clone remains unclear. The variable in vitro and in vivo efficacy of epigenetic drugs in DLBCL,[55,56] the predilection for *CREBBP* functional domain missense mutations in low-grade FL as opposed to truncating/frameshift mutations in DLBCL,[57] and an observed enrichment of *EZH2* mutation and amplification at transformation,[28,37] together support an ongoing and dynamic role for epimutations in aggressive disease. Furthermore, it is noteworthy that both *CREBBP* and *EZH2* mutation are associated with MHC downregulation,[51,54] given that immune evasion is considered an important mediator of HT. Meanwhile, transcriptomic heterogeneity has been suggested as an important driver of the phenotypic heterogeneity that enables cancer cells to undergo Darwinian tumor evolution.[58] It is feasible that epimutations contribute to an increased state of transcriptomic heterogeneity, laying a fertile soil for aggressive transformation, as well as or instead of targeting specific functional processes. A deeper understanding is required of the roles of epimutations individually and collectively, how these roles may evolve over different stages of disease, and the interaction with other genomic aberrations and the immune microenvironment. This process may in turn inform the use of emerging epigenetic-targeted drugs within the existing treatment repertoire.

CELL OF ORIGIN CLASSIFICATION AND HISTOLOGIC TRANSFORMATION

Alizadeh and colleagues's[59] seminal description of two transcriptionally defined DLBCL entities, GC B-cell (GCB) and activated B-cell subtypes, with different putative cell of origin and distinct clinical outcomes, has had significant bearing on both biological and clinical studies into de novo DLBCL. Although today this explanation may be an oversimplification, consistent at least with the pathologic and molecular GC phenotypic features of FL, the majority (70%–80%) of HT cases classify as GCB-DLBCL by gene expression profile.[16,34,60] The overall HT mutational landscape also equates to a GCB subtype,[27] with recurrent mutational targets including *EZH2* and *TNFRSF14*. However, a significant (approximately 20%) minority of cases classify as activated

B-cell subtype,[16,34] as reflected in the presence of NF-κB mutations both in low-grade FL (*TNFAIP3* and *CARD11*) and transformed FL (*MYD88*),[37] and intriguingly this group is also enriched for t(14;18) negativity.[16]

Meanwhile, although recent large-scale multiomic profiling efforts have sought to unravel the molecular heterogeneity of de novo DLBCL beyond the GCB/activated B-cell classification,[43–45] these studies have omitted HT cases, and thus a thorough analysis of where the observed heterogeneity of HT sits within the spectrum of DBLCL at the molecular level is lacking. As consensus emerges over the classification of novel DLBCL molecular subgroups, the cell of origin classification of HT deserves far greater attention, especially where subgroup-specific tailored treatments emerge.

ROLE OF THE IMMUNE MICROENVIRONMENT

There is now substantial evidence supporting the complementary crosstalk between the tumor cells and its microenvironment milieu. The landmark study from Dave and colleagues[61] describing 2 gene expression signatures, characterized by expression of T-cell (good prognosis) and macrophage-related (poor prognosis) gene sets, underlined the importance of the tumor microenvironment to outcomes in FL, albeit without examining the impact on transformation risk itself.

Indeed, only a minority of studies have related the tumor microenvironment to transformation specifically, with risk factors for future HT including intrafollicular localization of CD4$^+$ T cells[19,62,63] or CD14$^+$ follicular dendritic cells,[64] greater follicular infiltration with CD68$^+$/PD-L1$^+$ macrophages,[63] and greater microvessel density,[65] whereas data regarding CD21$^+$ follicular dendritic cell meshwork disruption[19,63,66] and FOXP3$^+$ T regulatory cell number and distribution[19,62,63,67,68] have been conflicting.

CD4$^+$ T-cell expression of the immune checkpoint programmed cell death protein 1 (PD-1) has received particular attention in light of the application of immune check point inhibition in a range of cancers. Recent studies are resolving early discrepancies regarding the prognostic significance of CD4$^+$ PD-1$^+$ T-cell numbers,[69–71] with diffuse/interfollicular, PD-1^{low} staining representing a TIM-3 coexpressing, exhausted T-cell population associated with greater transformation risk,[64,72] distinct from PD-1^{high} CXCR5$^+$ intrafollicular T follicular helper cells.[72]

Taken together, observations regarding the tumor microenvironment and transformation have been typically disparate, and not uncommonly contradictory. Immunohistochemical studies are hindered by a propensity to interobserver variability and their limited multiplexing ability, and heterogeneity in treatment regimens is considerable, with a number of the studies taken from the prerituximab era. Novel technologies, applied to well-defined cohorts, may help to resolve the contribution of immune populations to transformation biology, with time of flight mass cytometry proteomics,[73] single cell transcriptomics,[74] and highly multiplexed imaging approaches using heavy metal or nucleic acid-based antibody tagging,[75,76] beginning to emerge in FL and other cancers.

RECENT EFFORTS IN TRANSFORMATION PREDICTION

With the significant ongoing morbidity and mortality burden from HT, attention has rightly remained on efforts to predict those patients destined to transform, although clinically applicable progress has been modest thus far. The widely used baseline Follicular Lymphoma International Prognostic Index (FLIPI)[77] is predictive of transformation in prerituximab and postrituximab era datasets[5,6,18]—albeit without the sensitivity or specificity to alter management. Newer biological outcome predictors m7-FLIPI[78] (incorporating mutation status in *EZH2*, *ARID1A*, *MEF2B*, *EP300*,

FOXO1, *CREBBP*, and *CARD11* with FLIPI and Eastern Cooperative Oncology Group performance status) and a 23 gene expression-based signature[79] both hold promise for the refinement of upfront prognostication, but were not designed to predict HT specifically, nor have they been validated with this in mind.

An understanding of the dynamics of clonal evolution represents one potential route to the prediction of transformation. Although Kridel and colleagues[28] described the scarcity of the latter transformation clone in the initial FL biopsy in the majority of cases, casting some doubt on the ability to ever preempt transformation at diagnosis, this finding may at least partly reflect the mutational spatial heterogeneity in FL,[80] and thus highlights the limitations of the current single-site biopsy approach. Furthermore there was a minority (2 of 12 [13%]) of cases characterized as having only minor clonal evolution from diagnosis and less than 1 year to transformation, suggesting that a proportion of cases may indeed have features in the diagnostic biopsy from which to predict impending transformation[28]. This finding may have particular relevance given the inferior outcomes for those with early (within 18 months of diagnosis) transformation.[5] Indeed, the tendency for transformation rate to plateau after 5 to 15 years in at least some studies[1,2,5] would argue against a purely probabilistic model of ongoing transformation risk, and support the ongoing work to identify cases that may carry an inherent HT potential at diagnosis.

A broader tumor sampling afforded by circulating tumor DNA (ctDNA) analysis may increase the pick up of HT at diagnosis: Scherer and colleagues[81] observed that the dramatic clonal evolution reported from paired FL-HT biopsies[28], was also seen as an increased mutational divergence in the ctDNA mutational profile of cases with HT rather than indolent progression, forming the basis of an algorithm that was able to distinguish HT and indolent progression noninvasively.[81] They further described a case of HT where baseline ctDNA analysis was capable of detecting mutations that were absent in the diagnostic biopsy, but present in the HT biopsy 9 months later. Finally, their ctDNA analysis was able to predict HT (albeit at a modest average 66 days before clinical diagnosis), offering some encouragement of the potential of serial ctDNA sampling as a dynamic marker of evolving HT.

Transformation prediction at the gene expression level has been described in pre-rituximab datasets, with a signature akin to follicular hyperplasia,[19] and an embryonic stem cell-like gene expression program[39] predicting for HT. Brodtkorb and colleagues[82] described 6 predictive signatures associated with NF-κB pathway genes. Revisiting these 6 signatures in a single-agent rituximab-treated cohort, it was recently shown that the *BTK* signature consisting of 37 NF-κB target genes retained significance, combining with the FLIPI score to predict time to transformation and next treatment.[83] These data reaffirm the importance of NF-κB dysregulation to transformation in at least a proportion of cases. Overall, gene expression studies afford the opportunity to examine broader processes involved in transformation that may transcend the considerable genetic heterogeneity, and indeed may warrant renewed consideration in the context of improved NGS technologies, and modern treatment cohorts.

PET imaging has found a role in identifying HT at diagnosis, by guiding the choice of biopsy site to areas of discordant 18F-fluorodeoxyglucuose avidity. Regarding a role in prognostication, total tumor metabolic volume at diagnosis predicts for progression-free survival,[84] and end of treatment PET positivity predicts for both poorer progression-free survival and overall survival,[85,86] although a link between these parameters and future transformation risk specifically remains to be shown. Indeed a recent analysis of immunochemotherapy-treated FL patients from the GALLIUM study reported that higher baseline PET maximum standardized uptake value did not predict for subsequent biopsy-proven transformation, albeit with low numbers of transformed cases reported (13 of 522).[87]

SUMMARY

HT remains a poor prognostic event in the immunochemotherapy era, with only one-half of patients alive at 10 years after HT,[8] and represents an important area of ongoing research. A wealth of data has afforded us a landscape view of the processes involved in HT, with genome-wide NGS studies particularly pivotal in delineating the evolutionary dynamics and recurrent genomic events underpinning this critical disease-defining event. Stemming from these advances, ctDNA assessment holds considerable potential to help accomplish earlier identification of HT. Further progress requires ongoing reappraisal of the existing observations within an evolving therapy landscape and a renewed acknowledgment of the heterogeneity that may arise from the different clinical routes to transformation. Meanwhile, a clearer picture of the complex interplay between genetic lesions, epigenetic (dys)regulation, and the tumor microenvironment may unlock novel therapeutic opportunities. Although single cell resolution technologies, innovative bioinformatic approaches, and the development of authentic model systems may all play important roles, the inclusion of HT patients within trials of novel agents and accompanying biomarker discovery is imperative. The ultimate goal remains the translation of a deeper biological understanding into clinically actionable end points, which may include the early prediction of transformation, precision targeting of transformation-associated processes, or ultimately the prevention of transformation through early eradication of the founding FL CPC.

DISCLOSURE

Our research is supported by Cancer Research UK (15968 awarded to J. Fitzgibbon, 22742 awarded to J. Okosun) and Bloodwise program grant [15002] through the Precision Medicine for Aggressive Lymphoma (PMAL) consortium. E.A. Kumar is in receipt of fellowship funding from The Medical College of Saint Bartholomew's Hospital Trust. J. Fitzgibbon declares grants from Epizyme and personal fees from Roche, Gilead and Epizyme.

REFERENCES

1. Bastion Y, Sebban C, Berger F, et al. Incidence, predictive factors, and outcome of lymphoma transformation in follicular lymphoma patients. J Clin Oncol 1997; 15(4):1587–94.
2. Montoto S, Davies AJ, Matthews J, et al. Risk and clinical implications of transformation of follicular lymphoma to diffuse large B-cell lymphoma. J Clin Oncol 2007; 25(17):2426–33.
3. Al-Tourah AJ, Gill KK, Chhanabhai M, et al. Population-based analysis of incidence and outcome of transformed non-Hodgkin's lymphoma. J Clin Oncol 2008;26(32):5165–9.
4. Wagner-Johnston ND, Link BK, Byrtek M, et al. Outcomes of transformed follicular lymphoma in the modern era: a report from the National LymphoCare Study (NLCS). Blood 2015;126(7):851–7.
5. Link BK, Maurer MJ, Nowakowski GS, et al. Rates and outcomes of follicular lymphoma transformation in the immunochemotherapy era: a report from the

university of Iowa/mayo clinic specialized program of research excellence molecular epidemiology resource. J Clin Oncol 2013;31(26):3272–8.

6. Alonso-Álvarez S, Magnano L, Alcoceba M, et al. Risk of, and survival following, histological transformation in follicular lymphoma in the rituximab era. A retrospective multicentre study by the Spanish GELTAMO group. Br J Haematol 2017;178(5):699–708.

7. Federico M, Caballero Barrigón MD, Marcheselli L, et al. Rituximab and the risk of transformation of follicular lymphoma: a retrospective pooled analysis. Lancet Haematol 2018;5(8):e359–67.

8. Sarkozy C, Maurer MJ, Link BK, et al. Cause of death in follicular lymphoma in the first decade of the rituximab era: a pooled analysis of French and US cohorts. J Clin Oncol 2018. https://doi.org/10.1200/JCO.18.00400.

9. Swerdlow S, Campo E, Harria N, et al. WHO classification of tumours of haematopoietic and lymhpoid tissues. 4th edition. Geneva (Switzerland): World Health Organization; 2008.

10. Maeshima AM, Omatsu M, Nomoto J, et al. Diffuse large B-cell lymphoma after transformation from low-grade follicular lymphoma: morphological, immunohistochemical, and FISH analyses. Cancer Sci 2008;99(9):1760–8.

11. Rusconi C, Anastasia A, Chiarenza A, et al. Outcome of transformed follicular lymphoma worsens according to the timing of transformation and to the number of previous therapies. A retrospective multicenter study on behalf of Fondazione Italiana Linfomi (FIL). Br J Haematol 2019;185(4):713–7.

12. Wang Y, Farooq U, Link BK, et al. Late relapses in patients with diffuse large B-cell lymphoma treated with immunochemotherapy. J Clin Oncol 2019;37(21): 1819–27.

13. Swerdlow S, Campo E, Pileri S, et al. The 2016 revision of the World Health Organization classification of lymphoid neoplasms. Blood 2016;(127):2375–90.

14. Natkunam Y, Warnke RA, Zehnder JL, et al. Blastic/blastoid transformation of follicular lymphoma: immunohistologic and molecular analyses of five cases. Am J Surg Pathol 2000;24(4):525–34.

15. Thangavelu M, Olopade O, Beckman E, et al. Clinical, morphologic, and cytogenetic characteristics of patients with lymphoid malignancies characterized by both t(14;18)(q32;q21) and t(8;14)(q24;q32) or t(8;22)(q24;q11). Genes Chromosomes Cancer 1990;2:147–58.

16. Kridel R, Mottok A, Farinha P, et al. Cell of origin of transformed follicular lymphoma. Blood 2015;126(18):2118–27.

17. Macpherson N, Lesack D, Klasa R, et al. Small noncleaved, non-Burkitt's (Burkitt-Like) lymphoma: cytogenetics predict outcome and reflect clinical presentation. J Clin Oncol 1999;17(5):1558.

18. Giné E, Montoto S, Bosch F, et al. The Follicular Lymphoma International Prognostic Index (FLIPI) and the histological subtype are the most important factors to predict histological transformation in follicular lymphoma. Ann Oncol 2006; 17(10):1539–45.

19. Glas AM, Knoops L, Delahaye L, et al. Gene-expression and immunohistochemical study of specific T-cell subsets and accessory cell types in the transformation and prognosis of follicular lymphoma. J Clin Oncol 2007;25(4):390–8.

20. Lozanski G, Pennell M, Shana'ah A, et al. Inter-reader variability in follicular lymphoma grading: conventional and digital reading. J Pathol Inform 2013;4:30.

21. Ott G, Katzenberger T, Lohr A, et al. Cytomorphologic, immunohistochemical, and cytogenetic profiles of follicular lymphoma: 2 types of follicular lymphoma grade 3. Blood 2002;99(10):3806–12.

22. Koch K, Hoster E, Ziepert M, et al. Clinical, pathological and genetic features of follicular lymphoma grade 3A: a joint analysis of the German low-grade and high-grade lymphoma study groups GLSG and DSHNHL. Ann Oncol 2016;27(7): 1323–9.
23. Horn H, Schmelter C, Leich E, et al. Follicular lymphoma grade 3B is a distinct neoplasm according to cytogenetic and immunohistochemical profiles. Haematologica 2011;96(9):1327–34.
24. Horn H, Kohler C, Witzig R, et al. Gene expression profiling reveals a close relationship between follicular lymphoma grade 3A and 3B, but distinct profiles of follicular lymphoma grade 1 and 2. Haematologica 2018;103(7):1182–90.
25. Karube K, Guo Y, Suzumiya J, et al. CD10-MUM1+ follicular lymphoma lacks BCL2 gene translocation and shows characteristic biologic and clinical features. Blood 2007;109(7):3076–9.
26. Freeman CL, Kridel R, Moccia AA, et al. Early progression after BR is associated with high risk of transformation in advanced stage follicular lymphoma. Blood 2019;134(9).
27. Pasqualucci L, Khiabanian H, Fangazio M, et al. Genetics of follicular lymphoma transformation. Cell Rep 2014;6(1):130–40.
28. Kridel R, Chan FC, Mottok A, et al. Histological transformation and progression in follicular lymphoma: a clonal evolution study. PLoS Med 2016;13(12):1–25.
29. Rossi D, Cerri M, Paulli M, et al. Aberrant somatic hypermutation in transformation of follicular lymphoma and chronic lymphocytic leukemia to diffuse large B-cell lymphoma. Haematologica 2006;91:1405–9.
30. Correia C, Schneider PA, Dai H, et al. BCL2 mutations are associated with increased risk of transformation and shortened survival in follicular lymphoma. Blood 2015;125(4):658–67.
31. Yunis JJ, Frizzera G, Oken MM, et al. Multiple recurrent genomic defects in follicular lymphoma. A possible model for cancer. N Engl J Med 1987;316(2):79–84.
32. Tilly H, Rossi A, Stamatoullas A, et al. Prognostic value of chromosomal abnormalities in follicular lymphoma. Blood 1994;84(4):1043–9.
33. Eide MB, Liestøl K, Lingjærde OC, et al. Genomic alterations reveal potential for higher grade transformation in follicular lymphoma and confirm parallel evolution of tumor cell clones. Blood 2010;116(9):1489–97.
34. Bouska A, McKeithan TW, Deffenbacher KE, et al. Genome-wide copy-number analyses reveal genomic abnormalities involved in transformation of follicular lymphoma. Blood 2014;123(11):1681–90.
35. Elenitoba-Johnson KSJ, Gascoyne RD, Lim MS, et al. Homozygous deletions at chromosome 9p21 involving p16 and p15 are associated with histologic progression in follicle center lymphoma. Blood 1998;91(12):4677–85.
36. Sander CA, Yano T, Clark HM, et al. p53 Mutation is associated with progression in follicular lymphomas. Blood 1993;82(7):1994–2004.
37. Okosun J, Bödör C, Wang J, et al. Integrated genomic analysis identifies recurrent mutations and evolution patterns driving the initiation and progression of follicular lymphoma. Nat Genet 2014;46(2):176–81.
38. Lossos IS, Alizadeh AA, Diehn M, et al. Transformation of follicular lymphoma to diffuse large-cell lymphoma: alternative patterns with increased or decreased expression of c-myc and its regulated genes. Proc Natl Acad Sci U S A 2002; 99(13):8886–91.
39. Gentles AJ, Alizadeh AA, Lee SI, et al. A pluripotency signature predicts histologic transformation and influences survival in follicular lymphoma patients. Blood 2009;114(15):3158–66.

40. Musilova K, Devan J, Cerna K, et al. miR-150 downregulation contributes to the high-grade transformation of follicular lymphoma by upregulating FOXP1 levels. Blood 2018;132(22):2389–400.

41. Mottok A, Jurinovic V, Farinha P, et al. FOXP1 expression is a prognostic biomarker in follicular lymphoma treated with rituximab and chemotherapy. Blood 2018;131(2):226–35.

42. Akasaka T, Lossos IS, Levy R. BCL6 gene translocation in follicular lymphoma: a harbinger of eventual transformation to diffuse aggressive lymphoma. Blood 2003;102(4):1443–8.

43. Chapuy B, Stewart C, Dunford AJ, et al. Molecular subtypes of diffuse large B cell lymphoma are associated with distinct pathogenic mechanisms and outcomes. Nat Med 2018;24(5):679–90.

44. Reddy A, Zhang J, Davis NS, et al. Genetic and functional drivers of diffuse large B cell lymphoma. Cell 2017;171(2):481–94.e15.

45. Schmitz R, Wright GW, Huang DW, et al. Genetics and pathogenesis of diffuse large B-cell lymphoma. N Engl J Med 2018;378(15):1396–407.

46. Matolcsy A, Warnke R, Knowles D. Somatic mutations of the translocated bcl-2 gene are associated with morphologic transformation of follicular lymphoma to diffuse large-cell lymphoma. Ann Oncol 1997;8(Suppl 2):119–22.

47. Carlotti E, Wrench D, Matthews J, et al. Transformation of follicular lymphoma to diffuse large B-cell lymphoma may occur by divergent evolution from a common progenitor cell or by direct evolution from the follicular lymphoma clone. Blood 2009;113(15):3553–7.

48. Fitzgibbon J, Iqbal S, Davies A, et al. Genome-wide detection of recurring sites of uniparental disomy in follicular and transformed follicular lymphoma. Leukemia 2007;21(7):1514–20.

49. Weigert O, Kopp N, Lane AA, et al. Molecular ontogeny of donor-derived follicular lymphomas occurring after hematopoietic cell transplantation. Cancer Discov 2012;2(1):47–55.

50. Green MR, Gentles AJ, Nair RV, et al. Hierarchy in somatic mutations arising during genomic evolution and progression of follicular lymphoma. Blood 2013; 121(9):1604–11.

51. Green MR, Kihira S, Liu CL, et al. Mutations in early follicular lymphoma progenitors are associated with suppressed antigen presentation. Proc Natl Acad Sci U S A 2015;112(10):E1116–25.

52. Zhang J, Dominguez-Sola D, Hussein S, et al. Disruption of KMT2D perturbs germinal center B cell development and promotes lymphomagenesis. Nat Med 2015;21(10):1190–8.

53. Ortega-Molina A, Boss IW, Canela A, et al. The histone lysine methyltransferase KMT2D sustains a gene expression program that represses B cell lymphoma development. Nat Med 2015;21(10):1115–99.

54. Ennishi D, Takata K, Béguelin W, et al. Molecular and genetic characterization of MHC deficiency identifies ezh2 as therapeutic target for enhancing immune recognition. Cancer Discov 2019;9(4):546–63.

55. Knutson SK, Wigle TJ, Warholic NM, et al. A selective inhibitor of EZH2 blocks H3K27 methylation and kills mutant lymphoma cells. Nat Chem Biol 2012;8:890.

56. McCabe MT, Ott HM, Ganji G, et al. EZH2 inhibition as a therapeutic strategy for lymphoma with EZH2-activating mutations. Nature 2012;492(7427):108–12.

57. García-Ramírez I, Tadros S, González-Herrero I, et al. Crebbp loss cooperates with Bcl2 overexpression to promote lymphoma in mice. Blood 2017;129(19): 2645–56.

58. Hinohara K, Polyak K. Intratumoral heterogeneity: more than just mutations. Trends Cell Biol 2019;29(7):569–79.
59. Alizadeh AA, Eisen MB, Davis RE, et al. Distinct types of diffuse large B-cell lymphoma identified by gene expression profiling. Nature 2000;403(6769):503–11.
60. Elenitoba-Johnson KSJ, Jenson SD, Abbott RT, et al. Involvement of multiple signaling pathways in follicular lymphoma transformation: p38-mitogen-activated protein kinase as a target for therapy. Proc Natl Acad Sci U S A 2003;100(12):7259–64.
61. Dave SS, Wright G, Tan B, et al. Prediction of survival in follicular lymphoma based on molecular features of tumor-infiltrating immune cells. N Engl J Med 2004;351(21):2159–69.
62. Wahlin BE, Aggarwal M, Montes-Moreno S, et al. A unifying microenvironment model in follicular lymphoma: outcome is predicted by programmed death-1-positive, regulatory, cytotoxic, and helper T cells and macrophages. Clin Cancer Res 2010;16(2):637–50.
63. Blaker YN, Spetalen S, Brodtkorb M, et al. The tumour microenvironment influences survival and time to transformation in follicular lymphoma in the rituximab era. Br J Haematol 2016;175(1):102–14.
64. Smeltzer JP, Jones JM, Ziesmer SC, et al. Pattern of CD14+ follicular dendritic cells and PD1+ T cells independently predicts time to transformation in follicular lymphoma. Clin Cancer Res 2014;20(11):2862–72.
65. Farinha P, Kyle AH, Minchinton AI, et al. Vascularization predicts overall survival and risk of transformation in follicular lymphoma. Haematologica 2010;95(12): 2157–60.
66. Shiozawa E, Yamochi-Onizuka T, Yamochi T, et al. Disappearance of CD21-positive follicular dendritic cells preceding the transformation of follicular lymphoma: immunohistological study of the transformation using CD21, p53, Ki-67, and P-glycoprotein. Pathol Res Pract 2003;199(5):293–302.
67. Carreras J, Lopez-Guillermo A, Fox BC, et al. High numbers of tumor-infiltrating FOXP3-positive regulatory T cells are associated with improved overall survival in follicular lymphoma. Blood 2006;108(9):2957–64.
68. Farinha P, Al-Tourah A, Gill K, et al. The architectural pattern of FOXP3-positive T cells in follicular lymphoma is an independent predictor of survival and histologic transformation. Blood 2010;115(2):289–95.
69. Lopez-Guillermo A, Carreras J, Roncador G, et al. High numbers of tumor-infiltrating programmed cell death 1-positive regulatory lymphocytes are associated with improved overall survival in follicular lymphoma. J Clin Oncol 2009; 27(9):1470–6.
70. Muenst S, Hoeller S, Willi N, et al. Diagnostic and prognostic utility of PD-1 in B cell lymphomas. Dis Markers 2010;29(1):47–53.
71. Richendollar BG, Pohlman B, Elson P, et al. Follicular programmed death 1-positive lymphocytes in the tumor microenvironment are an independent prognostic factor in follicular lymphoma. Hum Pathol 2011;42(4):552–7.
72. Yang ZZ, Grote DM, Ziesmer SC, et al. PD-1 expression defines two distinct T-cell sub-populations in follicular lymphoma that differentially impact patient survival. Blood Cancer J 2015;5(2):e281.
73. Yang ZZ, Kim HJ, Villasboas JC, et al. Mass cytometry analysis reveals that specific intratumoral CD4 + T cell subsets correlate with patient survival in follicular lymphoma. Cell Rep 2019;26(8):2178–93.e3.

74. Milpied P, Cervera-Marzal I, Mollichella ML, et al. Human germinal center transcriptional programs are de-synchronized in B cell lymphoma. Nat Immunol 2018;19(9):1013–24.

75. Giesen C, Wang HAO, Schapiro D, et al. Highly multiplexed imaging of tumor tissues with subcellular resolution by mass cytometry. Nat Methods 2014;11(4): 417–22.

76. Goltsev Y, Samusik N, Kennedy-Darling J, et al. Deep profiling of mouse splenic architecture with CODEX multiplexed imaging. Cell 2018;174(4):968–81.e15.

77. Solal-Céligny P, Roy P, Colombat P, et al. FLIPI: follicular lymphoma international prognostic index. Blood 2004;104(5):1258–65.

78. Pastore A, Jurinovic V, Kridel R, et al. Integration of gene mutations in risk prognostication for patients receiving first-line immunochemotherapy for follicular lymphoma: a retrospective analysis of a prospective clinical trial and validation in a population-based registry. Lancet Oncol 2015;16(9):1111–22.

79. Huet S, Tesson B, Jais JP, et al. A gene-expression profiling score for prediction of outcome in patients with follicular lymphoma: a retrospective training and validation analysis in three international cohorts. Lancet Oncol 2018;19(4):549–61.

80. Araf S, Wang J, Korfi K, et al. Genomic profiling reveals spatial intra-tumor heterogeneity in follicular lymphoma. Leukemia 2018;32(5):1258–63.

81. Scherer F, Kurtz DM, Newman AM, et al. Distinct biological subtypes and patterns of genome evolution in lymphoma revealed by circulating tumor DNA. Sci Transl Med 2016;8(364):1–12.

82. Brodtkorb M, Lingjærde OC, Huse K, et al. Whole-genome integrative analysis reveals expression signatures predicting transformation in follicular lymphoma. Blood 2014;123(7):1051–4.

83. Steen CB, Leich E, Myklebust JH, et al. A clinico-molecular predictor identifies follicular lymphoma patients at risk of early transformation after first-line immunotherapy. Haematologica 2019;104(10):e460–4.

84. Meignan M, Cottereau AS, Versari A, et al. Baseline metabolic tumor volume predicts outcome in high-tumor-burden follicular lymphoma: a pooled analysis of three multicenter studies. J Clin Oncol 2016;34(30):3618–26.

85. Trotman J, Luminari S, Boussetta S, et al. Prognostic value of PET-CT after first-line therapy in patients with follicular lymphoma: a pooled analysis of central scan review in three multicentre studies. Lancet Haematol 2014;1(1):e17–27.

86. Trotman J, Barrington SF, Belada D, et al. Prognostic value of end-of-induction PET response after first-line immunochemotherapy for follicular lymphoma (GALLIUM): secondary analysis of a randomised, phase 3 trial. Lancet Oncol 2018;2045(18):1–13.

87. Mir F, Barrington SF, Meignan M, et al. Baseline Suvmax did not predict histological transformation from follicular lymphoma to aggressive lymphoma in the phase III GALLIUM study. Blood 2018;132(Supplement 1):4160.

Treatment of Histologic Transformation

Carla Casulo, MD

KEYWORDS

- Follicular lymphoma • Transformed lymphoma • Histologic transformation • Therapy
- Prognosis

KEY POINTS

- Histologic transformation of follicular lymphoma has improved outcomes.
- Novel approaches to treatment include chemoimmunotherapy and in some cases hematopoietic stem cell transplant or chimeric antigen receptor T-cell therapy.
- Ongoing research is exploring molecular and biological biomarkers contributing to the transformed phenotype.

INTRODUCTION

Follicular lymphoma (FL) represents the most common indolent non-Hodgkin lymphoma (NHL), affecting approximately 14,000 patients in the United States every year.[1] FL has a very long natural history and median overall survival (OS) exceeding 20 years; it is thought to be largely incurable based on patterns of frequent relapses throughout a patient's lifetime, despite long periods of disease control. The occurrence of histologic transformation to an aggressive lymphoma represents an important therapeutic and prognostic crossroad in a patient's trajectory and historically has been associated with poor outcomes. In the modern era, responses to chemotherapy, duration of response, and the opportunity for consolidation with high-dose chemotherapy and autologous stem cell transplant all seem to be altering the previous bleak landscape of this biological event. This review provides an overview of transformation of FL, diagnosis, and a review of some therapeutic options for patients with transformed disease.

DEFINITION OF HISTOLOGIC TRANSFORMATION

Histologic transformation (HT) refers to a biological evolutionary process whereby FL develops into a high-grade, aggressive NHL such as Burkitt lymphoma, high-grade B-cell lymphoma with translocations of *MYC* and *BCL2* (so called "double hit lymphoma"), lymphoblastic lymphoma, or more commonly, diffuse large B-cell lymphoma

Medicine and Oncology, Wilmot Cancer Institute, 601 Elmwood Avenue Box 704, Rochester, NY 14642, USA
E-mail address: Carla_Casulo@URMC.Rochester.edu

Hematol Oncol Clin N Am 34 (2020) 785–794
https://doi.org/10.1016/j.hoc.2020.03.001
0889-8588/20/© 2020 Elsevier Inc. All rights reserved.

hemonc.theclinics.com

(DLBCL). HT may occur with any indolent lymphoma, such as small lymphocytic lymphoma, marginal zone lymphoma, or lymphoplasmacytic lymphoma. However, for the purposes of this review the authors focus solely on HT of FL.

BIOLOGY OF TRANSFORMATION

The process of HT involves a rich vast array of genetic alterations and tumor evolution that is not limited to any singular biological event. Several genes are enriched on HT, either through activation of known oncogenes or inactivation of putative tumor suppressor genes, including *TP53*, *MYC*, *CDKN2A/B*, and *B2M*.[2] Parallel molecular disruptions leading to aberrant somatic hypermutation and copy number alterations result in a genomic landscape most similar to germinal center type DLCBL. Studies are ongoing to further determine whether the path to HT occurs more through a linear sequence of successive genetic events or through a process of divergent evolution. Further exploration of biological drivers and molecular mechanisms underlying HT in FL are discussed in greater detail in this series by Dr Jude Fitzgibbon.

INCIDENCE OF TRANSFORMATION

The reported incidence of HT derives mostly from retrospective series that differ in methodology. HT can be an early disease-related event, occurring frequently, but not always, within the first few years of diagnosis.[3–5] The risk ranges broadly from about 5.2% to 17% at 5 years, to approximately 20% to 30% at 10 years, with variability based on heterogeneity of therapy, treatment in the pre- and post-rituximab era, pathologic versus clinical evaluation, and surveillance strategies (**Table 1**).[4–9,11–14] As novel therapies for the first-line treatment of FL emerge, ongoing assessment of HT will be required, as these may change the natural history of FL.

Lack of consistent biopsies at the time of first progression or suspected HT hampers the true actuarial rate of HT in the literature. Two large contemporary studies in the rituximab era underscore the limited use of biopsies to confirm HT. Sarkozy and colleagues[5] evaluated risk factors and outcomes of patients with FL and HT after response to first-line chemoimmunotherapy with rituximab with cyclophosphamide, doxorubicin, vincristine, and prednisone (R-CHOP); rituximab with cyclophosphamide, vincristine, and prednisone; and rituximab with fludarabine, cyclophosphamide, and mitoxantrone in the Primary Rituximab and Maintenance Trial (PRIMA). Of 1108 patients, 464 experienced disease recurrence (45.5%), but of these, only 194 patients (42%) underwent a biopsy. HT was identified in 40 patients (20.6%) of those biopsied and in 8.6% of all those with disease progression. The median time to HT was 9.7 months from randomization in this series, but this excluded patients without a biopsy, biasing the true median time to HT.

Eleven cooperative groups across Europe pooled data on 10,001 patients with FL to assess the cumulative hazard of HT and survival after HT.[4] Patients enrolled from prospective clinical trials or hospital-/population-based registries and only those with biopsy confirmed HT as the first event following first-line systemic treatment was included. Patients were included if they had FL grade 1-3a as defined by the World Health Organization and diagnosed between1997 and 2003. Of 10,001 patients, 8116 were eligible for analysis. Among these, 4911 (60.5%) had disease progression. Of 4911 patients, 1012 (20.6%) underwent a biopsy. HT was identified in 509 patients (50.3%) of those biopsied and in 10.3% of all those with disease progression. Transformed diagnoses included DLBCL, FL grade 3b, lymphoblastic lymphoma, and Burkitt lymphoma. The cumulative hazard was 5.8% at 5 years and 7.7% at 10 years; median time from initial diagnosis to HT was 19 months.

Table 1
Comparison of incidence and frequency of histologic transformation

Reference/Author	Frequency/Incidence	Patient Details	Methodology	Plateau in Risk?	OS After HT	Impact of Treatment
Bastion et al,[14] 1997	24% incidence overall; 22% at 5 y; 31% at 10 y	34 patients, pre-rituximab era	Pathologic evaluation, clinical suspicion	Yes, after 6 y	Median OS 7 mo	NA
Montoto et al,[6] 2007	17% at 5 y, 28% at 10 y	186 patients, pre-rituximab era	Pathologic evaluation (73% had biopsy at first recurrence)	Yes, after 15 y	Median OS 1.2 y	Expectant management predicted for higher risk of HT
Al-Tourah et al,[7] 2008	3% per year, 30% at 10 y	170 patients, pre-rituximab era	Pathologic evaluation, clinical suspicion	No plateau	5-y OS 25%	No difference in HT risk based on initial treatment
Link et al,[8] 2013	10% at 5 y, 2% per year	60 patients, rituximab era	Pathologic evaluation (85%), clinical suspicion	Slowed after 5 y (short follow-up)	Median OS 50 mo	HT risk higher in patients initially observed
Wagner-Johnson et al,[9] 2015	6% at 2 y, 10.9% at 4 y, 19% at 8 y	379 patients, rituximab era	Pathologic evaluation, clinical suspicion	NA	Med OS post-HT 5-y OS from diagnosis 75%	Treatment at diagnosis had reduced risk of HT, maintenance R associated with reduced HT
Sarkozy et al,[5] 2016	4.1% at 6 y	40 patients, rituximab era	Pathologic evaluation, clinical suspicion	NA	Median OS 3.8 y	NA
Garvin et al,[10] 1983	32% incidence	192 patients, pre-rituximab era	Autopsy	NA	NA	NA
Bains et al,[11] 2013	18% at 5 y	11 patients, early-stage disease, rituximab era (mix)	Pathologic evaluation, clinical suspicion	NA	10-y OS 50%	NA
Conconi et al,[12] 2012	15% at 10 y	37 patients, rituximab era (mix)	Pathologic evaluation	NA	37% at 5 y, 13% at 10 y	Treatment increased the risk of HT
Federico et al,[4] 2018	10-y Hazard 7.7%	509 patients, rituximab era (mix)	Pathologic evaluation	NA	10-y OS after HT 32%	Treatment was associated with decreased risk of HT
Alonso-Alvarez et al,[13] 2017	8% at 10 y	106 patients, mostly non-rituximab treated	Pathologic evaluation	NA	5-y OS 26%	No difference in HT with treatment or observation

Data from Refs.[4–8,10–15]

RISK FACTORS FOR TRANSFORMATION

The use of rituximab as a routine part of lymphoma therapy seems to have altered the natural history of FL and in some series, the risk of subsequent transformation as well. Several prospective studies established rituximab as a standard of care, given improved response rates and OS when used alone and in combination with chemotherapy.[16–19] As part of a maintenance strategy, long-term follow-up from the PRIMA study shows that maintenance rituximab for 2 years following rituximab/chemotherapy also prolongs progression-free survival (PFS).[20] Whether use of rituximab (alone or with chemotherapy) actually decreases the risk of HT is a matter of controversy, with inconsistent results depending on the series. Sometimes the risk is unknown or not reported.[10,14] A population-based series from Al-Tourah and colleagues[7] from British Columbia (BC) in the pre-rituximab era reported no difference in the risk of HT based on initial treatment, and an analysis from the prospective multicenter F2 study found no increased HT risk in patients with FL undergoing watchful waiting.[21] In a Swiss report by Conconi and colleagues,[12] the incidence of HT was significantly increased in patients initially managed with rituximab/chemotherapy and reduced in those managed initially expectantly. In a single institution series from BC, Freeman and colleagues[3] note that following bendamustine-based therapy, patients with FL with an early recurrence were enriched for transformed disease in about 75% of cases, although biopsies were not uniformly performed. In contrast, several other groups have noted a decrease in the reported frequency of HT based on use of rituximab/chemotherapy at the time of first-line therapy compared with observation.[6,8,15] Clinical risk factors such as high Follicular Lymphoma International Prognostic Index score,[5] the presence of extranodal sites and elevated lactate dehydrogenase (LDH),[5,15,22] advanced stage, older age, poor performance status, and higher histologic grade[5,12] are more prevalent in transformed cases and seem to contribute to risk.

IDENTIFYING HISTOLOGIC TRANSFORMATION

The gold standard in identifying HT involves an excisional biopsy whenever possible. This permits adequate study of the lymph node architecture for appropriate grading. Furthermore, it facilitates additional cytogenetic evaluation if suspecting transformation to a high-grade B-cell lymphoma with translocations of *MYC* and *BCL2*, which may alter choice of next therapy. A core biopsy would be an acceptable alternative if an excisional biopsy is not feasible, but a fine-needle aspirate is almost never acceptable, given limited size of the specimen; unless patient condition, disease site or other factors impede preferable diagnostic measures. As noted in prior studies,[4,20] rates of biopsy to prove HT at the time of FL recurrence are low and depend largely on physician preference, patient condition, and suspicion of transformed disease. There seems to be no difference in outcomes when HT is diagnosed based on laboratory values (elevated LDH, hypercalcemia, new extranodal sites of disease) or biopsy.[7,8]

A PET scan can be useful in identifying hypermetabolic disease sites harboring higher-grade lymphoma. In independent studies by Schöder[23] and Ngeow,[24] increased SUV_{max} was observed in patients with aggressive NHL compared with indolent NHL, with a cutoff of SUV_{max} of 10 yielding a sensitivity ranging between 71% and 91% and a specificity between 62% and 81% to identify aggressive disease. Noy and colleagues[25] looked specifically at PET in transformed lymphomas, noting the median SUV in a PET scan from transformed lymphoma of 12, with half of cases presenting with SUV_{max} greater than 13.

INITIAL TREATMENT AND PROGNOSIS OF HISTOLOGIC TRANSFORMATION

Approach to therapy for HT is variable and depends on whether or not a patient is treatment naïve and if not, the type of treatment received for prior indolent lymphoma. There are no prospective studies guiding therapy, and most recommendations emerge from retrospective series. Historical data report dismal outcomes of HT, particularly in the pre-rituximab era, where median OS ranged from 1 to 2 years.[11,14,26,27] However, more contemporary data incorporating rituximab demonstrate promising survival, comparable to de-novo DLBCL. These contemporary studies lend hope to the prognosis of HT in the modern era. In the largest of these, Wagner-Johnson and colleagues report outcomes of 379 patients from the National LymphoCare Study treated in the rituximab era. Diagnoses were made both on clinical grounds and with pathologic evaluation. Of patients with HT, 5-year OS was inferior when compared with patients without HT (75% OS vs 85% OS; 95% confidence interval, 83–86). Median posttransformation OS was 4.9 years. When comparing patients initially observed or treated, and anthracycline-based treatment versusnonanthracycline-based treatments, no difference in OS posttransformation was observed.[15] Likewise, among 77 patients with HT at the time of diagnosis (composite histology), both PFS and OS at 5 years were similar when compared with patients without HT (66% vs 61% and 88%, respectively). Treatment patterns following HT varied, and few patients received consolidation with autologous stem cell transplant (ASCT).

Ban-Hoefen and colleagues[28] analyzed 118 patients with HT of FL in the National Comprehensive Cancer Network (NCCN) database treated in the rituximab era. Patients were included if diagnosed between 2000 and 2011 and received several first-line therapies including observation in a small subset and chemotherapy/chemoimmunotherapy. OS at 2 and 5 years was 68% and 49%, respectively. However, survival of patients naïve to prior chemotherapy before HT was superior when compared with patients exposed to chemotherapy before HT (100% vs 35%, $P = 0.03$).

In the University of Iowa and Mayo Clinic experience, patients with HT had survival similar to patients with de novo DLBCL, with an OS of 66% at 5 years.[8] However, median OS was longer in those who transformed later than 18 months from diagnosis versus those with HT within 18 months of diagnosis (66% vs 22%; $P<.001$). Consistent with outcomes by Ban-Hoefen and colleagues, patients who received R-CHOP before transformation had inferior outcomes compared with those receiving R-CHOP at the time of HT (OS at 5 years, 21% vs 66%; $P<.001$). Only 8 patients received ASCT for consolidation after HT. Similar outcomes were observed in registry data from the Royal Marsden experience and the Spanish GrupoEspañolde Linfoma y Transplante Autólogode Médula Ósea (GELTAMO) group (5-year OS of 64% and 55%, respectively, following R-CHOP),[13,29] most of whom did not receive ASCT as consolidation. Patients without prior treatment of FL in the GELTAMO series had superior 5-year posttransformation OS compared with those who were treated (44% vs 24%; $P = .16$), although numbers were small (n = 9).

Interpretation of these data suggests that first-line treatment of transformed disease in an anthracycline-naïve patient (either rituximab only or no prior treatment) should consist of standard R-CHOP. R-CHOP would also be reasonable if HT is present at diagnosis. In a recent analysis of the University of Iowa and the Mayo Clinic, patients with concurrent DLBCL and other indolent lymphomas (composite or discordant lymphoma or considered as early transformation of a previously undiagnosed indolent lymphoma) had similar event-free survival and OS (hazard ratio [HR] = 1.09) when compared with patients with DLBCL alone.[30]

Patients with high-grade B-cell lymphoma and cytogenetic rearrangements of *MYC*, *BCL2*, and/or *BCL6* may be treated with more aggressive strategies such as dose-adjusted etoposide, prednisone, vincristine, cyclophosphamide, and doxorubicin. However, patients who received prior anthracycline-based therapy should be approached similarly to relapsed DLBCL and be considered for salvage therapy and consolidation with ASCT.

AUTOLOGOUS STEM CELL TRANSPLANT IN THE RITUXIMAB ERA

Studies investigating the role of ASCT sought to improve the historically poor outcomes observed in the pre-rituximab era. This body of literature supports high-dose therapy and ASCT consolidation for patients with chemosensitive disease, resulting in 5-year PFS and OS rates of 32% and 47%.[31] However, the highly selected, generally younger patient population included in these small studies poses a challenge to generalization. Given the current standard of chemoimmunotherapy as first-line therapy for FL, the position of ASCT within the treatment paradigm is relevant and requires reevaluation.

The largest report of ASCT for transformed disease was published by the Canadian Blood and Marrow Transplant Group where 97 received ASCT and 57 were treated with chemoimmunotherapy.[32] There was a modest benefit in OS and PFS of patients with ASCT compared with chemoimmunotherapy (5-year OS of 65% with ASCT; 61% with rituximab and chemotherapy; HR = 0.13; $P<.001$), and in multivariate analysis, ASCT was an independent predictor of favorable outcome (HR = 0.13; $P<.001$).

In the NCCN database, 2-year OS was 83% with ASCT. However, patients younger than 60 years without prior rituximab exposure receiving chemoimmunotherapy only and not undergoing ASCT also had very promising outcomes, with 5-year OS of 80%.[28]

A retrospective Danish study by Madsen and colleagues investigated ASCT in 85 patients with HT, of whom 54 (64%) underwent ASCT. The remaining patients received chemoimmunotherapy. When compared with chemoimmunotherapy, ASCT did not seem to improve OS or PFS if HT was found at the time of diagnosis, although it did improve the outcome of patients with HT following diagnosis (termed sequential transformation). At 5 years, OS was 62% versus 36% ($P = .07$) and PFS 53% versus 6% ($P = .002$) regardless of prior rituximab therapy. The beneficial effect of ASCT was also significantly higher in patients who had not received rituximab as part of first-line treatment.[33]

Other smaller studies demonstrate 5-year OS and PFS ranging between 60% and 70% and 40% and 45%, respectively, when ASCT is used as part of the therapy strategy (**Table 2**). Collectively, the data suggest the benefit of ASCT in HT may be greatest when used as part of a second-line treatment strategy in patients when used earlier in the treatment course (second-line) and when used in younger patients. The authors' strategy is to use ASCT in the appropriate fit patient who has had prior chemoimmunotherapy for indolent lymphoma and chemosensitive disease following second-line therapy.

CHIMERIC ANTIGEN RECEPTOR T-CELL THERAPY

For aggressive B-cell lymphomas refractory to or relapsing after first-line therapy, anti-CD19 chimeric antigen receptor (CAR) T cells have emerged as a promising treatment therapy, resulting in durable remissions in up to 40% of patients. There are currently 2 Food and Drug Administration (FDA)-approved anti-CD19 CAR T-cell products, axicabtageneciloleucel (axi-cel) and tisagenlecleucel (tisa-cel), both of which have

Table 2
Studies of autologous stem cell transplant in the rituximab era

Study	N	OS (%)	PFS or EFS (%)
Reddy et al,[35] 2012	51	62% at 5 y	45% at 5 y
Ban-Hoefen et al,[28] 2013	50	83% at 2 y	N/A
Ban-Hofen et al, 2012	18	82% at 2 y	59% at 2 y
Villa et al,[32] 2013	97	65% at 5 y	55% at 5 y
Smith et al,[34] 2009	25	64% at 3 y	59% at 3 y
Madsen et al,[33] 2015	65	65% at 5 y	57% at 5 y

Data from Refs.[28,32–35]

been studied in HT. The pivotal study using axicabtagenecicloleucel included 16 patients with transformed FL. Overall response rate (ORR) was 83% and duration of response was 11 months.[36] Schuster and colleagues[37] studied the use of tisagenlecleucel in 21 patients with HT. ORR was 52%, and durable responses have been observed for up to 18 months following treatment. CAR T-cell therapy can be considered in a patient with persistent disease following 2 lines of therapy (FDA-approved indication).

ALLOGENEIC TRANSPLANT

Literature describing allogeneic transplant (allo-SCT) in HT reports modest survival benefit and high rates of treatment-related mortality (TRM). OS at 4 to 5 years ranges between 20% and 68%, TRM of about 25%, and graft versus host disease affecting nearly half of patients. Allo-SCT may provide long-term survival in select patients who are younger and have fewer therapeutic options available.[32]

TARGETED AGENTS

Although used increasingly less often, radioimmunotherapy has historical relevance in the treatment of HT.[31] [131]Itositumomab (Bexxar) and ^{90}Y-ibritumomab tiuxetan (Zevalin) have been promising treatments for HT, both as part of ASCT and alone. ORR ranges between 39% and 79%, with 50% complete response (CR), and median response duration of 3 years.[38]

A paucity of data on HT in prospective studies limits information on efficacy of novel therapies. One phase II study did test the immunomodulator lenalidomide in patients with HT showing an ORR of 57% and median response duration of greater than 1 year.[39] In combination with rituximab, Wang and colleagues[40] from MD Anderson Cancer Center reported ORR of 33% and median response duration of 10.2 months.

FUTURE DIRECTIONS

New therapeutic targets are currently being studied in patients with relapsed DLBCL that may be considered in HT. In June 2019, the FDA approved polatuzumab vedotin in combination with bendamustine plus rituximab for the treatment of patients with relapsed/refractory DLBCL after at least 2 prior lines of treatment. Polatuzumab vedotin is an antibody-drug conjugate against CD79b, part of the B-cell receptor complex. Although not currently approved for transformed lymphoma, this agent has an ORR of 50% when combined with bendamustine/rituximab.[41] Future studies may be testing polatuzumab-based combinations in the transformed setting.

Interim analysis of the bispecific antibody against CD3/CD20, mosunetuzumab, was recently presented at the 2019 annual meeting of the American Society of Hematology. Thirty-two patients with transformed lymphoma were included. Of these, 8 patients had been previously treated with anti-CD19 CAR T-cell therapy. ORR was 37%, and CR was 19%. Mosunetuzumab combinations are being further evaluated in the front-line and relapsed settings and seem to be promising for patients with HT.[42]

SUMMARY

HT had previously been a rare but devastating clinical development in the natural history of FL, with poor outcomes. Current use of first-line chemoimmunotherapy has changed this prognosis, and patients with HT at time of diagnosis or subsequent relapse now have greater therapeutic options that may offer long-term disease control.

Given lack of prospective studies guiding treatment selection, the best available evidence must be weighed against patient condition and prior therapy. The development of other novel treatments including next-generation anti-CD20 antibodies, targeted drugs, and biologics will continue to expand the therapeutic landscape for patients with HT.

REFERENCES

1. Teras LR, DeSantis CE, Cerhan JR, et al. 2016 US lymphoid malignancy statistics by World Health Organization subtypes. CACancer J Clin 2016;66(6):443–59.
2. Kridel R, Chan FC, Mottok A, et al. Histological transformation and progression in follicular lymphoma: a clonal evolution study. PLoS Med 2016;13:e1002197.
3. Freeman CL, Kridel R, Moccia AA, et al. Early progression after bendamustine-rituximab is associated with high risk of transformation in advanced stage follicular lymphoma. Blood 2019;134:761–4.
4. Federico M, Caballero Barrigon MD, Marcheselli L, et al. Rituximab and the risk of transformation of follicular lymphoma: a retrospective pooled analysis. LancetHaematol 2018;5:e359–67.
5. Sarkozy C, Trneny M, Xerri L, et al. Risk factors and outcomes for patients with follicular lymphoma who had histologic transformation after response to first-line immunochemotherapy in the PRIMA trial. J ClinOncol 2016;34:2575–82.
6. Montoto S, Davies AJ, Matthews J, et al. Risk and clinical implications of transformation of follicular lymphoma to diffuse large B-cell lymphoma. J ClinOncol 2007; 25:2426–33.
7. Al-Tourah AJ, Gill KK, Chhanabhai M, et al. Population-based analysis of incidence and outcome of transformed non-Hodgkin's lymphoma. J ClinOncol 2008;26:5165–9.
8. Link BK, Maurer MJ, Nowakowski GS, et al. Rates and outcomes of follicular lymphoma transformation in the immunochemotherapy era: a report from the University of Iowa/MayoClinic Specialized Program of Research Excellence Molecular Epidemiology Resource. J ClinOncol 2013;31:3272–8.
9. Wagner-Johnson N, Link B, Taylor M. Risk Factors for Early Transformation of Follicular Lymphoma (FL): Report From the National LymphoCare Study (NLCS). Blood 2009;114(22):2698.
10. Garvin AJ, Simon RM, Osborne CK, et al. An autopsy study of histologic progression in non-Hodgkin's lymphomas. 192 cases from the National Cancer Institute. Cancer 1983;52:393–8.

11. Bains P, Al Tourah A, Campbell BA, et al. Incidence of transformation to aggressive lymphoma in limited-stage follicular lymphoma treated with radiotherapy. Ann Oncol 2013;24:428–32.

12. Conconi A, Ponzio C, Lobetti-Bodoni C, et al. Incidence, risk factors and outcome of histological transformation in follicular lymphoma. Br J Haematol 2012;157: 188–96.

13. Alonso-Alvarez S, Magnano L, Alcoceba M, et al. Risk of, and survival following, histological transformation in follicular lymphoma in the rituximab era. A retrospective multicentre study by the Spanish GELTAMO group. Br J Haematol 2017;178:699–708.

14. Bastion Y, Sebban C, Berger F, et al. Incidence, predictive factors, and outcome of lymphoma transformation in follicular lymphoma patients. J ClinOncol 1997;15: 1587–94.

15. Wagner-Johnston ND, Link BK, Byrtek M, et al. Outcomes of transformed follicular lymphoma in the modern era: a report from the National LymphoCare Study (NLCS). Blood 2015;126:851–7.

16. Hainsworth JD, Litchy S, Burris HA 3rd, et al. Rituximab as first-line and maintenance therapy for patients with indolent non-hodgkin's lymphoma. J ClinOncol 2002;20:4261–7.

17. Marcus R, Imrie K, Belch A, et al. CVP chemotherapy plus rituximab compared with CVP as first-line treatment for advanced follicular lymphoma. Blood 2005; 105:1417–23.

18. Luminari S, Ferrari A, Manni M, et al. Long-term results of the FOLL05 trial comparing R-CVP versus R-CHOP versus R-FM for the initial treatment of patients with advanced-stage symptomatic follicular lymphoma. J ClinOncol 2018;36(7): 689–96.

19. Rummel MJ, Niederle N, Maschmeyer G, et al. Bendamustine plus rituximab versus CHOP plus rituximab as first-line treatment for patients with indolent and mantle-cell lymphomas: an open-label, multicentre, randomised, phase 3 non-inferiority trial. Lancet 2013;381:1203–10.

20. Bachy E, Seymour JF, Feugier P, et al. Sustained progression-free survival benefit of rituximab maintenance in patients with follicular lymphoma: long-term results of the PRIMA study. J ClinOncol 2019;37:2815–24.

21. Solal-Celigny P, Bellei M, Marcheselli L, et al. Watchful waiting in low-tumor burden follicular lymphoma in the rituximab era: results of an F2-study database. J ClinOncol 2012;30:3848–53.

22. Conconi A, Franceschetti S, Aprile von Hohenstaufen K, et al. Histologic transformation in marginal zone lymphomasdagger. Ann Oncol 2015;26:2329–35.

23. Schoder H, Noy A, Gonen M, et al. Intensity of 18fluorodeoxyglucose uptake in positron emission tomography distinguishes between indolent and aggressive non-Hodgkin's lymphoma. J ClinOncol 2005;23:4643–51.

24. Ngeow JY, Quek RH, Ng DC, et al. High SUV uptake on FDG-PET/CT predicts for an aggressive B-cell lymphoma in a prospective study of primary FDG-PET/CT staging in lymphoma. Ann Oncol 2009;20:1543–7.

25. Noy A, Schoder H, Gonen M, et al. The majority of transformed lymphomas have high standardized uptake values (SUVs) on positron emission tomography (PET) scanning similar to diffuse large B-cell lymphoma (DLBCL). Ann Oncol 2009;20: 508–12.

26. Yuen AR, Kamel OW, Halpern J, et al. Long-term survival after histologic transformation of low-grade follicular lymphoma. J ClinOncol 1995;13:1726–33.

27. Advani R, Rosenberg SA, Horning SJ. Stage I and II follicular non-Hodgkin's lymphoma: long-term follow-up of no initial therapy. J ClinOncol 2004;22:1454–9.
28. Ban-Hoefen M, Vanderplas A, Crosby-Thompson AL, et al. Transformed non-Hodgkin lymphoma in the rituximab era: analysis of the NCCN outcomes database. Br J Haematol 2013;163:487–95.
29. Gleeson M, Hawkes EA, Peckitt C, et al. Outcomes for transformed follicular lymphoma in the rituximab era: the Royal Marsden experience 2003-2013. LeukLymphoma 2017;58:1805–13.
30. Wang Y, Link B, Witzig T, et al. Impact of concurrent indolent lymphoma on the clinical outcome of newly diagnosed diffuse large B-cell lymphoma. Blood 2019;134:1289–97.
31. Casulo C, Burack WR, Friedberg J. Transformed follicular non-Hodgkin lymphoma. Blood 2015;125:40–7.
32. Villa D, Crump M, Panzarella T, et al. Autologous and allogeneic stem-cell transplantation for transformed follicular lymphoma: a report of the Canadian blood and marrow transplant group. J ClinOncol 2013;319:1164–71.
33. Madsen C, Pederson MB, Vase MO, et al. Outcome determinants for transformed indolent lymphomas treated with or without autologous stem-cell transplantation. Ann Oncol 2015;2:393–9.
34. Smith S, Bolwell BJ, Advani AS, et al. High rate of survival in transformed lymphoma after autologous stem cell transplant: pathologic analysis and comparison with de novo diffuse large B-cell lymphoma. LeukLymphoma 2009;50:1625–31.
35. Reddy N, Oluwole O, Greer J, et al. Superior long-term outcome of patients with early transformation of non-Hodgkin lymphoma undergoing stem cell transplantation. Clin Lymphoma Myeloma Leuk 2012;126:406–11.
36. Neelpau S, Locke F, Bartlett N, et al. Axicabtageneciloluecel CAR T-cell therapy in refractory large B-cell lymphoma. N Engl J Med 2017;26:2531–44.
37. Schuster S, Bishop M, Tam CS, et al. Tisangenlecleucel in adult relapsed or refractory diffuse large B-cell lymphoma. N Engl J Med 2019;380:45–56.
38. Zelenetz AD, Saleh M, Vose J. Patients with transformed low grade lymphoma attain durable responses following outpatient radioimmunotherapy with tositumomab and iodine I 131 tositumomab (Bexxar). Blood 2002;100:357a [abstract].
39. Czuczman M, VoseJ, Witzig T, et al. The differential effect of lenalidomidemonotherapy in patients with relapsed or refractory transformed non-Hodgkin lymphoma of distinct histological origin. Br J Haematol 2011;154:477–81.
40. Wang M, Fowler N, Wagner-Bartak N, et al. Oral lenalidomide with rituximab in relapsed or refractory diffuse large cell, follicular and transformed lymphoma: a phase II clinical trial. Leukemia 2013;9:1902–9.
41. Sehn LH, Herrera AF, Flowers CR, et al. Polatuzumabvedotin in relapsed or refractory diffuse large B-cell lymphoma. JClinOncol 2020;38:155–65.
42. Schuster SJ, Bartlett NL, Assouline S, et al. Mosunetuzumab induces complete remissions in poor prognosis non-hodgkin lymphoma patients, including those who are resistant to or relapsing after chimeric antigen receptor T-cell (CAR-T) therapies, and is active in treatment through multiple lines. ASH Annual Meeting Abstracts. San Diego, 2020.

Moving?

Make sure your subscription moves with you!

To notify us of your new address, find your **Clinics Account Number** (located on your mailing label above your name), and contact customer service at:

Email: journalscustomerservice-usa@elsevier.com

800-654-2452 (subscribers in the U.S. & Canada)
314-447-8871 (subscribers outside of the U.S. & Canada)

Fax number: 314-447-8029

Elsevier Health Sciences Division
Subscription Customer Service
3251 Riverport Lane
Maryland Heights, MO 63043

*To ensure uninterrupted delivery of your subscription, please notify us at least 4 weeks in advance of move.